Reiki

A Complete Steps From Basic to Master Level

(The All-in-one Reiki Manual for Deep Healing and Spiritual Growth)

Ralph Carlson

Published By **Regina Loviusher**

Ralph Carlson

Reiki: A Complete Steps From Basic to Master Level (The All-in-one Reiki Manual for Deep Healing and Spiritual Growth)

ISBN   978-1-998769-89-6

Legal & Disclaimer

The information contained in this ebook is not designed to replace or take the place of any form of medicine or professional medical advice. The information in this ebook has been provided for educational & entertainment purposes only.

The information contained in this book has been compiled from sources deemed reliable, and it is accurate to the best of the Author's knowledge; however, the Author cannot guarantee its accuracy and validity and cannot be held liable for any errors or omissions. Changes are periodically made to this book. You must consult your doctor or get professional medical advice before using any of the

TABLE OF CONTENTS

Chapter 1: Understanding Reiki

Reiki is a herbal restoration approach from Japan. Universal lifestyles strength, as Reiki is known as, is transferred by using laying on of fingers. Anyone can exercise Reiki. All you want to do is attend a seminar with a Reiki master. The ubiquitous life strength can then be handed on more concentrated. Reiki is used nowadays now not handiest in Japan, however additionally in different nations in hospitals as an adjunctive remedy. It is likewise broadly used in many recovery practices and for treating your self, family and buddies. Scientific research have tested its effectiveness. The WHO has recognized Reiki as an alternative therapy. Find out on this book what Reiki is, the way it works, in which you may learn it, and how a Reiki remedy works.

What is Reiki?

Coming from Japan, Reiki is a machine that via the direct or oblique imposition of fingers, permits electricity to be channeled from the Universe to the patient through their chakras or power facilities, permitting them to harmonize and balance their physical, emotional, intellectual body.

Reiki is a Japanese shape of the laying on of fingers and one of the oldest natural recovery methods. The purpose of the treatment is to convey frame, soul and spirit into harmony and to discover a religious path to oneself.

Reiki is a safe, holistic herbal healing therapy, because it treats the human being as an entire, easy to apply and can deal with many acute and persistent ailments, together with allergies, rhinitis, cystitis, chronic fatigue, sinusitis, arthritis, sciatica, depression, insomnia, sell non secular, intellectual and emotional well-being. It is appropriate for anyone, with out regulations.

It is an exceptional tonic. If you are in suitable bodily situation, reiki will help you live that manner.

Reiki is a gentle, lively approach wherein electricity is transferred and the self-healing powers to be activated. To do this, arms are placed at the body in positive positions for several mins. Reiki has no constant aim. The Reiki giver is a channel for the popular energy, which also can be referred to as divine strength. He passes it on and the frame of the Reiki recipient makes use of it as it needs it. Both humans do not interfere with their will. This additionally applies to lengthy-distance and intellectual remedies.

It is not one's personal strength that flows, in any other case the transmission would be laborious. Instead, by means of giving Reiki, one is supplied with this power and feels empowered. The laying on of hands is thought in all cultures. Every mother intuitively lays her hand on the kid while a infant is injured, and one does it mechanically in the event of abdominal ache or different lawsuits. Reiki only amplifies the energy this is flowing.

Reiki, which in Japanese method accepted power, consists of channeling through the arms a effective supply of vibration, that is out of doors, closer to oneself or towards other humans to heal physical illnesses or heal feelings. In addition, absolutely everyone can exercise or acquire it, because it isn't a special gift reserved for the privileged few, however as an alternative a method that may be discovered.

Alternative Therapies work from the idea that every one physical contamination originates in the first example within the thoughts or in the emotions, and that the person should have the actual preference to heal, turning into the principle protagonist in their recovery procedure and ceasing to be affected person but as an alternative active in this system.

Reiki postulates that by means of recovery the Spirit and the emotional beyond, we are able to heal our frame and circulate toward religious development, towards the state of Satori or Enlightenment, and stay the search for a country of calm and perfect concord, regardless of what happens to us.

From the point of view of Alternative Therapies, illness is a direction, a first rate Master who constantly involves educate us something, an enjoy in our lives thru which we've the possibility to research. When we come to be protagonists of our personal healing manner and take fee of the moves which could have a right away have an effect on at the pain we experience, at that particular second, it's far that we will get right of entry to the healing and improvement of our infection.

And it's miles exactly at this factor in which Reiki has the opportunity of bringing the affected person closer to full cognizance and harmonization, even if the character does not trust in it and irrespective of their religious traits, because it acts independently in their opinions and beliefs. In addition, Reiki does not want units, it has no contraindications nor does it have any conflict with tablets or other remedies, however instead it tends to reduce the facet consequences that they could be causing.

Those therapists who have a more superior level of Reiki also can ship it remotely and with unique symbols that allow directing the goal in keeping with the want of the person who has asked it, and also can use those symbols to send this healing energy to some past trauma that has left an power blockage and that might presently be inflicting an infection.

The exciting element is that the therapist is most effective a channel, and the reality of having been initiated in Reiki permits him to be a bridge between the regular power and the affected person, ruling out any possibility of switch of poor energies or fatigue that the therapist should have at the moment to perform the Reiki session.

Those who work with Reiki additionally exercise every day the 5 fundamental standards that were delivered by way of its discoverer, the Japanese Mikao Usui, which lets in them to get right of entry to everlasting non secular boom and that with practice will increase the go with the flow of energy that they could channel, allowing get right of entry to to new gear and a excessive improvement of instinct or clairvoyance, which is also more suitable with the aid of using a series of strategies to smooth aura, environments, harmonize chakras, etc.

It must be noted that there are a series of Reiki Systems created each in the West and within the East from the unique System but whose final intention refers -via the manner- to same goal that its creator expressed and which might be summarized in those five splendid principles:

1. Just for nowadays don't worry

2. Just for today do not be indignant

three. Honor your dad and mom, teachers and elders

four. Earn your livelihood definitely

five. Show gratitude for the whole thing that surrounds you

Therefore, it does not rely what kind of Reiki someone applies, but rather that they do it with the actual purpose of healing themselves and coming across that past the bodily comfort, there is a spirit that is crying out for help, and that it is time to hear it.

How was Reiki Discovered?

Reiki changed into taught with the aid of Dr. Mikao Usui (1865-1926), a Japanese monk and essential of a Christian college in Kyoto. In seek of a technique that might heal the frame and mind, Dr. Usui studied Buddhist, Christian and different scriptures for years, traveled to distinct international locations and in the end retired for 21 days to fast return. In doing so, he found out how he may want to use energy as a restoration force. He founded the primary Reiki medical institution, practiced and taught the technique in the course of Japan. After his loss of life, his college students, along with Dr. Hayashi continued his work.

In 1935, Hawayo Takata, daughter of Japanese who had emigrated to Hawaii, made her way to

Japan looking for a therapy for her bodily illnesses. At the Reiki Clinic in Tokyo, she recovered absolutely. She became a Reiki grasp and taken the approach to america. From there, she got here to Europe. Among other Reiki masters, Takata additionally educated her granddaughter Phyllis Furumoto, who after the dying of her grandmother has held her function as grand grasp to these days.

How Does Reiki Work?

Reiki combines historic healing traditions with current, scientific fashions. Our bodies are obviously lively. Your bones vibrate at a low frequency, even as your blood and thoughts, as an example, vibrate at a higher frequency. This magnetic pulse is referred to as the bio-magnetic area.

The principle is that after humans carry out Reiki, they act as a type of link between the individual being treated and the source of established existence pressure electricity at that second. The strength flows thru the arms of the man or woman doing the remedy into the frame of the person being dealt with.

The man or woman to be handled determines the drift of electricity that flows via the hands via best accepting the part of it that they need. It allows the affected person realize that we're most effective assisting them with what they want and not with what we suppose they want. This is an appropriate stability to meet the wishes of the affected person.

When you lay for your arms, you may experience the acute flow of power thru warmth. The nice, rather powerful strength penetrates the entire body. Blockages and tensions are launched. Circulation and metabolism are inspired. The body is purified and detoxified. And not only the frame, but additionally poor thought styles and emotions, resentment and fears may be launched. The foremost feeling is deep rest. It appears to penetrate to the ultimate mobile. This deep relaxation isn't always simplest appropriate for you. It has a restoration effect on stress harm, lowers blood strain and intellectual and religious high anxiety, relieves ache, relieves cramps, improves sleep and promotes the healing system.

Trust and self-confidence are strengthened; the coronary heart is opened, and all this with out exceptional charges and with out side consequences. What can show are cleansing reactions: tears that have been suppressed for a long time can drift once more, antique reviews come to thoughts once more and can be easily processed, the frame detoxifies with corresponding smells. Reiki may be utilized in aggregate with another healing technique. In the event of contamination, it does now not replace a visit to the medical doctor or naturopath.

Doctors have developed gadgets which can measure the bio-magnetic field. Measuring this subject regularly presents higher information approximately the nation of fitness of a person and what goes on of their body than conventional electronic measurements.

When a Reiki practitioner conducts a Reiki session, the energy emanating from their fingers creates a miles large bio-magnetic reading than does a non-practitioner. This cost is round 7-10 Hz and is therefore in the theta and alpha variety. These frequencies are associated with physical recovery. After a Reiki treatment, human beings may additionally experience:

• Satisfaction

• Relaxation

• Reduced emotions of strain, tension and restlessness

• Reduction and in a few instances even elimination of bodily ailments and continual ailments

These observations are documented and confirmed by using numerous medical empirical research and case studies. So Reiki is not a way that you have to believe in for it to work. In 2007, Reiki was even identified as an opportunity restoration approach by using the World Health Organization.

Origin

The Japanese monk Mikao Usui (1865-1926) developed Reiki as a system of non secular exercise that mixes knowledge and techniques from one-of-a-kind traditions. Healing is said to be effected thru the usage of symbols, used like talismans, and through the laying on of arms. Influences from Buddhism, Taoism and Tibetan scriptures can be visible in Reiki. There is a legend approximately the emergence of the healing orientation of religious practice this is often repeated by using Usui's followers.

Mikao Usui is said to have located 2,500-yr-antique Tibetan sutras written in Sanskrit that explained the healing effects of laying on of palms using Reiki symbols. Usui turned into satisfied that he had found the healing technique that Jesus Christ is stated to have used to carry out his brilliant healings. However, no such Tibetan sutras are acknowledged to this point, and Usui himself is mentioned to have said that the Reiki symbols are original.

Not knowing a way to interpret those Reiki symbols, Usui retreated to Japan's Mount Kuriyama for meditation, wherein after 3 weeks of fasting and meditating, he had a imaginative and prescient. The following morning, he struck his foot on a stone, bleeding. When Usui positioned his fingers at the wound, the bleeding stopped. On the identical day, he was able to therapy a female of toothache. So Usui started to heal human beings together with his arms and later to train the Reiki method.

Usui's scholar Chijiro Hayashi (1879-1940) wanted to develop a healing approach from spiritual exercise and based the primary private Reiki clinic in Tokyo round 1930 after Usui's demise. Hayashi's successor Hawayo Takata (1900-1980) in turn made Reiki internationally recognized from Hawaii. Until her death in 1980, she initiated 22 Reiki masters to pass on her knowledge.

Takata's granddaughter Phyllis Furumoto is now diagnosed by means of many Reiki masters because the Grand Master of the Usui machine. She founded the Reiki Alliance and teaches in 3 tiers with approximately 5 signs. Barbara Ray, who turned into also initiated by Takata, questions Furumoto's legitimacy as Takata's successor and claims the identify of Grandmaster for herself. In her own corporation, modern-day The Radiance Technique Association International (TRTAI), she teaches with seven ranges and about 30 characters. Today, there are Reiki directions, with Furumoto's Usui system being the most popular in Europe.

Basics

According to the Reiki philosophy, contamination and stress stand up whilst a person's connection to the common life energy is blocked. For instance, because of long-suppressed emotions. Reiki followers expect that everybody is usually born with the capability to take in and skip in this popular life electricity. However, if you want to use them in a centered manner, preparation from a Reiki master or teacher is required, who will initiate the pupil. Special seminars are offered for this reason, in which the diverse Reiki levels may be discovered.

The Reiki master or trainer acts as a mediator who transmits the familiar lifestyles energy to the scholar. This strengthens the life energy of the student and promotes the self-recuperation energy of his frame. Reiki calls for normal practice and paintings on oneself from the scholar; relying on the Reiki stage achieved, he stories a better degree of attention.

The Reiki concept includes the view that life electricity handiest flows where there is a need for it. Likewise, an excessive amount of energy cannot be transferred from the Reiki grasp to the recipient, in view that best as an awful lot electricity is absorbed as is absolutely wished. The more electricity flows for the duration of a treatment, the more the blockage or lack of electricity inside the corresponding strength area. In addition, according to the Reiki practitioners, the power of the grasp himself is by no means transmitted, but he most effective opens a channel for the patient in order that he can acquire the life electricity once more.

History

A younger priest desired to discover how Jesus healed and discovered Reiki. The story of the Reiki founder Dr. Mikao Usui is the story of a quest that ended luckily. Usui devoted his lifestyles to answering this question.

Reiki is set Dr. Mikao Usui

Dr. Mikao Usui was head of a small university in Kyoto and at the same time a clergyman. The query of whether he changed into of the Christian faith is disputed. Dr Usui left university and went to the united states to take a look at ancient languages in Chicago. He wanted with a view to examine the texts of historic information strategies inside the authentic. He discovered that Buddha had additionally possessed the strength of recuperation.

Returning to Japan, Usui searched monasteries for the solution to how healing by way of hands works. There he observed little help because the monasteries had been busy recuperation the spirit and now not interested in recuperation the bodily frame. Eventually he stayed in a Zen monastery and studied the sutras, Buddhist texts that deal substantially with preventive health measures. He discovered symbols and the outline of ways Buddha had healed within the statistics.

Dr. Usui believed he had reached his aim due to the fact he had rediscovered the antique knowledge. However, he soon found out that he nonetheless lacked the electricity to heal. He turned into convinced that the solution should simplest lie in meditation, so he went to the holy mountain Kurama for twenty-one days to rapid and meditate. After twenty days, he nevertheless hadn't found a solution, however then a vivid beam of light flooded him and knocked him to the floor, a satori moment. He noticed the symbols he already knew in bubbles of light.

How and for what's reiki utilized in aggregate with conventional medication?

In addition to Japan, more and more other countries are offering Reiki in hospitals and clinical practices, in particular inside the USA and Great Britain. In Germany, Reiki is used, for example, in the Charité Berlin. Indications are pre-op and post-op care, inclusive of for the duration of operations, accompanying cancer, AIDS, acute infections, continual illnesses, in emergency remedy and infertility. Positive outcomes are stress discount, ache remedy, acceleration of recovery and rehabilitation, much less use of medicine, fewer side effects of medicine, improvement of urge for food and sleep.

Dr. Usui Believes He Has Reached His Goal

On the way lower back, he injured his foot, so he couldn't stroll any in addition. Gripping the bleeding foot with both fingers, the pain and bleeding subsided quick, and he turned into able to hold on his manner. On the same day, he healed a woman from excessive toothache and shortly afterwards his pal the abbot of the Zen monastery from an assault of arthritis. His strength to heal turned into now so strong that he may want to treatment sufferers with just one treatment. For the subsequent seven years, Dr. Usui in a slum in Japan, he helped many people to conquer illness and to enhance their state of affairs drastically.

Physical Healing is not Enough

After a few years, however, he turned into dismayed to find that a huge percentage of the humans he had healed were in the same awful circumstance as before. At first there was no explanation, however then he found out that even though he had healed the bodily body, he could not alternate the attitude towards life. People lacked gratitude, the notice that they had been satisfactory. As a end result, Dr. Usui pass after individuals who have been really inquisitive about a change and had been also thankful. He gave them the 5 Reiki rules of lifestyles.

Reiki Reduces Stress and Anxiety

Reiki is a so-referred to as energetic healing technique, that may sell relaxation and decrease strain and anxiety via mild touch. Mikao Usui evolved Reiki in the early 1900s. The term Reiki refers back to the critical lifestyles energy that flows thru all living matters. Today, Reiki is used in hospitals and hospices round the sector to complement other forms of remedy.

Healing Through Energetic Balance

Reiki can aid in recuperation by way of assisting human beings reap active stability — bodily, emotionally, mentally, and spiritually. Experts are convinced that the unique shape of treatment can make contributions to relaxation, pressure discount and relief of symptoms and enhance general health and well-being.

Reiki can also have a number of exceptional high quality outcomes on the body and mind, along with:

• Inducing a meditative state.

• Supporting recovery after accidents or operations.

• Stimulation of the immune machine.

• Promotion of the natural self-recovery powers.

• Relief of ache and anxiety.

• Improving the intellectual fitness of human beings undergoing traumatic medical treatments (radiation, chemotherapy, surgery and kidney dialysis).

Safety and Well-being Through Reiki

A 2019 look at also showed that Reiki instills a sense of peace, rest, security, and nicely-being.

Can Reiki Replace Conventional Treatments?

According to at least one expert, Reiki ought to not be used instead for scientific advice or psychotherapy, however complements other medical and therapeutic treatments and can beautify the effectiveness of different healing techniques. In wholesome humans, normal Reiki treatment also can improve the capacity to address stress and serve as a form of preventative remedy.

Because Reiki works on the whole self, i.E. Mind, frame and emotions and because it's far ordinary lifestyles energy, Reiki may be a success in all types of physical, emotional, mental and spiritual recuperation.

Reiki isn't always designed mainly for any precise type of infection or circumstance, but it is able to assist human beings with plenty of illnesses, which includes:

• Cancer.

• Chronic pain.

• Infertility.

• Digestive troubles.

• Parkinson's sickness.

• Psychological problems (e.G. Melancholy and anxiety).

• Diseases as a result of strain.

Reiki also can help people put together for upcoming surgeries. This makes it feasible for the restoration to be expanded after the operation.

Chapter 2: Reiki Principles Of Life

Reiki is an lively restoration exercise that originated in Japan. However, we find Reiki energy beneath one-of-a-kind names in lots of different traditions and cultures. In Germany, Reiki is likewise on occasion utilized in hospitals.

The Buddhist monk Mikao Usui (who's typically taken into consideration to be the founding father of Reiki) noticed the Reiki principles as the important thing to a happy lifestyles and referred to as them remedy for the soul.

Dr Usui taught 5 principles that may assist to integrate Reiki into one's own existence on the level of mind. These principles can help combine Reiki into your existence and come to be a pure channel for life strength. These ideas have been at first laid down with the aid of the Meiji Emperor of Japan (1868-1912) as guidelines for a fulfilling existence.

As I understand it, those suggestions have to never be taken as difficult and speedy rules, but can function a reminder to remember of one's thoughts and emotions. In this respect, they may be regarded as a stepping stone or an exercise in inner attention. Unfortunately, it is clean to misconceive these standards or take them as tough and speedy rules that risk suppressing or coercing positive thoughts or emotions. Rather, see these standards as some thing to be aware of on your normal existence and during your Reiki exercise.

The Deceptive Simplicity of the Reiki Principles

These ideas are the teachings of Usui, which have become some thing just like the roots of the Reiki machine. Its deceptive simplicity undermines its expertise and the difficulty of training and dwelling it every day.

The ideas themselves are corresponding to intentions or affirmations. It's approximately focusing at the here and now. They inspire us to embody the Reiki energy all through the day.

They speak about the significance of residing each day.

When the guidelines are significantly labored with, they now not become desires to be accomplished, however come to be incorporated into the action of each second and become a sort of subconscious law. As Usui wrote preceding the rules, they may be: The Secret Art of Inviting Happiness & the Spiritual Medicine for All Diseases.

In the following sections, I even have explained the Reiki rules of life in detail for you and give you a private assessment of how to interpret the regulations and use them for yourself.

No Strict Rules

As in all spiritual practices, I comply with an undogmatic approach to Reiki. I suppose there are a number of misunderstandings around the principles. I understand them in this sort of manner that they provide assist to integrate Reiki on a non secular level in ordinary existence. For me, however, they're no longer to be understood as strict policies, but as an alternative as a reminder of how we may be careful with our moves, mind and emotions.

If they are visible as strict policies, feelings inclusive of frustration or fear may be suppressed, which can result in strength pent-up and eventual blockages. There are several variations of the Reiki standards. So those are not a definitive list.

Negative Wording

There are increasing conversations that the Reiki ideas are formulated negatively. In principle, you may reformulate the Reiki rules of lifestyles for yourself.

For instance, I additionally recognize the bad formulations and feature chosen those fine ones (see underneath) due to the fact they are right for me. Since I additionally use quite a few affirmations in meditation, it's miles critical for me to paintings with fantastic formulations. It is entirely up to you how you need to combine the Principles into your life.

Positively Worded Reiki Affirmations

Just these days:

- Be free from anger

- Be unfastened from issues

- Be high-quality on your fellow humans

- Earn your residing actually

- Be thankful

The 5 Reiki Rules of Life

1. Don't agonize

2. Don't worry

three. Be grateful

4. Work tough (earn your dwelling genuinely)

five. Be type to the ones around you

1. Don't Fret

It's the first line, just these days, that gives immediacy to the regulations. Therefore, even though they may be known as the 5 regulations, there are virtually six commandments. Because that first line, simply these days, is perhaps the most critical of all of the guidelines to live through.

We interpret the time period in particular today in any such way that space and time do no longer exist and we honestly simplest stay in the here and now (these days) and may best achieve something there.

Experiencing anger isn't always always a bad aspect. It signals to us that a person or some thing may additionally have crossed a line. What sincerely subjects is how we address that anger. Get to the foundation and cause of the motive instead of blindly reacting to it.

This principle is a reminder that anger is authorized to surface and dissolve in its personal time, in preference to judging it or blaming us for it, which handiest permits anger to linger longer than essential. Feelings like anger show us that something isn't going in line with our desires or plan.

A plan offers avoidable control, in case you permit cross of manipulate, electricity can glide freely once more. I combine this point in any such manner that I do not suppress feelings like anger or frustration, however alternatively be given and face them with the aid of being mindful of my emotions and feelings.

I often ask myself, in which does this feeling come from, what does it want to inform or display me and the way can I specific it in order that it may transform and I can permit move of it.

Anger is not inherently incorrect and this recommendation must not be taken to intend that being irritated is a bad element. Anger and feelings are greater of a form of indication that some thing does not correspond to our expectations and needs. Anger, like all emotion, is a shape of life force energy this is now and again expressed in very uncooked and crude methods. Consciously handling anger can consequently be very high quality for dealing with different people, within the experience that we do not try and unload our anger on others and accordingly best begin a wildfire that in the end falls lower back on ourselves.

Mindful viewing of anger can transform those emotions; that is the name of the game of consciousness. Mindfulness is like internal alchemy. Raw gross power like anger and sexual power are transformed into finer better energies like love and compassion. But each person who has tried to remain aware all through a tantrum is aware of how difficult this emotion is to govern, and so it is every now and then helpful to use positive meditation techniques (e.G. Dynamic Meditation or the Pillow Hitting Meditation) to release the pent-up suppressed anger to let them act out in a kind of catharsis, a willful act of feelings without affecting other humans.

We recognise how hard this emotion is to govern and therefore it's far once in a while useful to apply sure meditation strategies (e.G. Dynamic meditation or the pillow-slapping meditation) to release the pent-up suppressed anger in a sort of catharsis, a inclined acting out of the emotions without the opposite human beings get hit via it. Of course, Reiki is likewise perfect for dealing with anger by clearly treating your self with Reiki in the sort of state of affairs.

Tip: When you sense anger arising, put one hand on your 3rd chakra/sun plexus (channel of anger) and one in your 4th chakra/heart chakra (channel of affection) and consciously breathe inside and outside. I sense into the anger and marvel in which it's miles coming from and what message it has for me. After that, it normally resolves itself and I come into gratitude.

2. Don't Worry

Unfortunately, it is not the case that our efforts and no longer trying to fear could mean that we would now not fear in a clearly tough situation (if for example, our accomplice or a relative is significantly sick). But many of our normal concerns are ultimately unfounded.

Researchers have determined that ninety nine% of the matters we worry approximately will in no way manifest. Ultimately, worry additionally stems from a preference with a view to manage and predict our destiny in order to give us some experience of protection.

Reiki gives us a tool in our palms with which we cannot most effective calm ourselves down and give a sense of security in ourselves, Reiki, much like meditation, brings us back to our basic trust. We have often forgotten what it is want to feel one with the universe, with lifestyles, or whatever you need to name it.

Reiki and meditation are not anything but methods that help us to rediscover our authentic state, which is simply there all the time. Only our trained concept styles, issues and fears hold us from feeling our proper nature. Everything we desire for from the lowest of our hearts, inclusive of love, joy, freedom, safety, oneness and happiness, are nothing other than manifestations of our natural kingdom of being.

Make up your thoughts and recognise that annoying approximately the future handiest method you suffer two times. Fears approximately the destiny are created within the now, however have nothing to do with our real future truth. This Reiki principle grounds you in the right here and now. Again, I don't take it that I need to never worry again, however that worries are simply the absence of consider.

In normal existence, constantly try to be aware about the connection, the relationship to the prevalent strength, to the universe and to everybody. Worries are either inside the beyond or in the future, I try to be greater present in regular life, meditation also enables me loads.

Through Reiki, we connect to the accepted power aka conventional love this is usually flowing in and via us. Where there is love, there may be consider and in which there's trust, there can be no sorrow.

Tip: Concentrate on the root chakra in the Reiki self-remedy and as a result toughen self-confidence and accept as true with.

3. Be Thankful for All Your Blessings

This precept is set presence in the ordinary moments that we basically velocity past. This is the present of a gratitude practice, receiving again appreciation for our ordinary lives.

Sometimes in our lives, we revel in short moments of happiness, love, freedom or unexpected perception into the mysteries of the universe. We see a starry sky, a flower momentarily feels deep fulfilment; from time to time we have a stunning interpersonal or sexual come upon, or we revel in a Reiki utility that brings us deep relaxation, relaxation or even touches us deeply. And yet we frequently skip via such activities carelessly and without appreciation, we take them with no consideration and cross immediately on with our everyday lives.

Such experiences are like an extraordinary guest in our house and if we meet this guest with pleasure, openness, appreciation and gratitude, then it's going to certainly be glad to visit us extra regularly. So is our dating with the

Universe, only whilst we are open and appreciative of the gifts we every so often receive, then the Universe is aware of it's far a welcome visitor in our home. The mystic Rumi as soon as stated, the entirety you are searching for seeks you. This means that if you stretch out your hand openly, the universe will possibly unknown to you, provide you its benefits.

But practicing gratitude manner no longer most effective surely appreciating the beautiful moments, but also developing an growing information of the importance of tough, difficult moments in life. They can continually see an occasion in their existence as a problem, i.E. Misfortune as a challenge, as an possibility or whilst a gift. It all depends on our evaluation and our angle.

The best crises in existence often end up the best items for our internal growth and adulthood. A tree this is never challenged by using the wind has no purpose to expand deep and strong roots. But it is precisely these sturdy, massive roots that supply it energy and power for even extra storms and additionally for its endured boom.

Through Reiki, we get a great deal extra grateful in regular lifestyles and celebrate the small rituals and combine them with gratitude. For instance, when I mild a candle, I deliver thank you for a feeling that I want to cultivate.

When we feature a stone on ourselves, we thank it for its positive effect, when we are in nature, we thank it for the colors, the clean air, and so on. It's greater about going through life and all its sides with gratitude and recognize the little matters in everyday life.

Just while we ask ourselves what we are grateful for without giving a solution, the chemistry in our brain adjustments, so it's so powerful to integrate gratitude into normal existence.

As a final word, saying thanks would not have to be something you do because it allows you or as it's a social habit. It should not be a hole phrase, a hollow gesture. Then it is honestly worthless.

Gratitude is some thing that comes to you more regularly whilst you apprehend the laws of the universe. If you apprehend how critical demanding situations are for you and what sort of you are on occasion talented. When you begin giving something to different people, as an example Reiki, you'll speedy realise which you are regularly the one who has to mention thanks, now not the one to whom you gave Reiki. Because you get what you deliver back, often lots of instances over. All of this gives you an increasingly more frequent and deepening feeling of gratitude.

4. Work Hard (on yourself)

This precept is about residing authentically and in your essence. It's about receiving abundance on your lifestyles without lying, dishonest, judging or manipulating to get in advance.

Since the entirety is strength, I also accept as true with that others can feel the power with which I perform a piece. For example, if I provide a meditation or record one, I always first bring myself into the mood that I need to ship out. By the manner, we do that with (almost) everything. If I experience terrible or frustrated, I prefer to take a damage until the feelings are neutralized once more.

This rule arguably relates primarily to internal spiritual practice, our day by day exercising in meditative attention. It simply would not suggest that we must work twelve hours hard to be glad or fulfilled. I think that is considered one of the most important misunderstandings in our subculture and additionally in Japanese way of life that many people, at the least for us, are simply starting to wake up to. Working hard interior doesn't suggest it's hard, it is extra like willpower and a willingness to stand up to yourself.

Because despite the fact that we acquire Reiki, supply Reiki to ourselves or to others, there's someplace the willingness to do some thing for oneself. It isn't usually smooth to offer loving attention to your self, through which I additionally mean your personal frame, mind, feelings, desires, and so forth. Apparently it's miles less complicated to distract yourself in the beginning. At some factor, we will be thrown returned on ourselves one way or every other, glad is the only who has used his existence to prepare for those stages in lifestyles. Of direction, Reiki is a way to do some thing precise for your self and others, to harmonize your self internally.

But once in a while you have to cross a chunk via the dust and garbage that has accrued over the years till you could breathe a sigh of alleviation and spot the sector in unheard of beauty. Our lifestyles strength is occasionally also like a cleansing hearth that internally burns the whole lot that is antique and superfluous and creates area for brand spanking new lifestyles. This can now and again be hard, however it constantly will pay off a thousand fold. Meditation is the country that brings us back to lifestyles refreshed and glad, just like a deep Reiki remedy, it reconnects us with our internal source.

The supply that is at the equal time the universal supply of all existence and all power, all consciousness. Mediation is doing not anything, just being. But to get into this kingdom calls for strategies for a protracted part of our religious route. Like a boat that you take to the other side, most effective if you have arrived does it make feel and is critical to leave the boat behind, to carry it on would be pointless ballast. But till then, a boat, this is, a method, is really important. In addition to its effect at the body and thoughts, Reiki is likewise a technique to get in contact with the internal nation of being, i.E. With meditation.

5. Be Kind to Those Around You

Being type and loving is lovely. But where does a loving, appreciative mind-set towards other people come from? The natural order to be kindly holy loving has often been shown in the beyond in the superimposed loving behavior with which Christians in particular have committed horrible crimes against youngsters and destroyed different cultures in missionary zeal. No person who loves himself can hate different people and do violence to them. Love and compassion begins with love and compassion for yourself.

The courting you have with yourself affects each person else. Reiki gives me the opportunity to be loving with myself, to spend a second simply with me, to do some thing exact for myself and to strengthen the connection with myself and deliver it new expression.

If I am glad and glad, this electricity is routinely transferred to my surroundings and how I address my fellow humans. So Reiki is the high-quality element I can provide myself and my fellow humans.

I believe that after I do something with poor electricity or vibes, the people my paintings reaches feel it. And if I'm satisfied with what I'm doing, that resonates in my work. In addition, we are able to most effective be glad and content material while we do paintings that fulfills us.

Of route, a positive well mannered way is beneficial for a functioning cooperation, but if the form is supposed to hide the real inner country of thoughts, simply so that the etiquette and the picture we need to offer to the out of doors global is to be maintained, then I would say it is better to select to be who you are right now. At the identical time, you may revel in that it's okay not to be satisfactory on occasion. This is useful when one desires to receive all components of 1's internal existence. This popularity is prime and precedes self-love and consequently attractiveness and love for other human beings. In order to be best and to our fellow human beings, we should begin with ourselves and be excellent to ourselves, then being high-quality to our fellow human beings will follow clearly.

But how can we be kind to ourselves, loving to ourselves?

Reiki is a wonderful way to be kind and loving to yourself. Do some thing precise in your body, do some thing exact in your head and do something excellent for your coronary heart. When you give yourself Reiki, you not only deliver your self life electricity however also interest and love. All of that is very restoration and you'll quick observe the way it has a effective effect for your properly-being and your dealings with other human beings. That's it for the 5 Reiki ideas of life.

Chapter 3: Getting Started With Reiki Treatment

You may have encounter Reiki at the same time as studying a way to loosen up and manipulate stress. Because further to alternative recovery methods which include acupuncture, acupressure, modern muscle relaxation, Reiki is a remedy that is becoming increasingly more popular.

Reiki, the time-honored existence energy, is contained in all living things. When a person becomes ill, their body indicates power deficits. He develops signs and symptoms that can be handled with a Reiki application. The electricity creation belongs to the sphere of holistic energy work and is obtainable these days by using many naturopaths in addition to in health clinics and well-being facilities.

In Reiki remedy, the practitioner only serves as a channel for the transmission of Reiki to the patient (purchaser). According to Reiki teachings, every form of contamination is as a result of lively blockages and energy deficits. The typical lifestyles energy can not go with the flow unhindered.

Certain regions of the body are energetically undersupplied as a end result. There are proceedings in cells, organs and complete body areas. Reiki dissolves the blockage at the nice-material stage. The aches and pains depart. The treatment, wherein frame, mind and soul are understood as a unit, does now not require a conventional prognosis and assumes that Reiki robotically finds the location inside the energetically ill body where it's far urgently wished.

Reiki works regardless of the affected person's mental kingdom. It has a nice impact on folks who are open to it and inclined to make the important adjustments in their lives. The health-selling effect is even greater if the Reiki person has a high degree of sensitivity. Scientific research at the effectiveness of Reiki treatment have no longer yielded any clean outcomes to date. With the assist of Reiki, the educated person may even treat himself, animals and plants.

What Happens in Reiki?

According to the unique teachings of Reiki, an infection arises from the imbalance of energies, whether or not on a physical, emotional and mental level. The laying on of fingers is supposed to channel and modulate existence electricity. The law of nature, the balancing of excess and deficiency are used right here. Reiki does no longer make any diagnoses! It helps the recovery and remedy methods of traditional and natural medicine. It does no longer replace the physician or naturopath.

Function, Effect & Goals

With Reiki, a distinction is made among short-term treatment for acute health disorders and full-frame treatments. They are generally performed within the case of significant persistent illnesses and really demanding symptoms.

Short remedies last up to 30 minutes. In the case of full treatments, the patron ought to reckon with a treatment time of up to at least one and a half hours. He is in a relaxed role on a mat on the ground. He is clothed due to the fact the standard strength can of route input his body through his apparel. The Reiki practitioner determines the lively state of his chakras (power centers) through laying his fingers on his forehead for 15 minutes. Then he puts his hand on the other chakras, shifting the power to them. Alternatively, the Reiki practitioner also can preserve his hand a few centimeters above the frame. Then the patron lies on his front in order that the again of the frame can be energetically treated.

From the individual chakras, the strengthening and restoration conventional energy is also handed directly to different components of the body. According to Mikao Usui, the discoverer of Reiki, the Reiki practitioner can also even lightly stroke, tap and rubdown the client's frame. The practitioner comes to a decision in line with the desires of the sick person. The

Reiki treatment impacts all subtle degrees. The harmonization of the mental and emotional kingdom promotes the bodily recuperation process. However, the affected person need to expect the preliminary aggravation impact to occur. In the case of acute issues, it is therefore beneficial to perform the remedy for 4 consecutive days in order that recovery occurs.

The initial aggravation is simply evidence that the remedy is effective and the body is prepared to reply to it. In the case of extreme psychological pressure, there may additionally initially be an emotional boost. It also indicates that the strength furnished causes adjustments. It is normally active five to 7 days after treatment.

In the case of chronic and extreme lawsuits, numerous packages are vital. On a mental and non secular stage, the widespread existence strength has the subsequent consequences: reduction of strain, merchandising of relaxation, increasing attention and studying capability, harmonization and intensification of the emotional lifestyles, letting cross of bad and hindering thought structures, advertising of internal power and composure, strengthening of creativity, intellectual flexibility, instinct, promotion of cognitive approaches (self-attention, reputation of one's personal cause in lifestyles), development of the mental and intellectual capacity, possibly promoting of religious capabilities.

Depressive moods and consuming disorders also are undoubtedly influenced by means of Reiki. The remedy need to now not be used in the presence of neuroses and psychoses. On a bodily stage, Reiki causes a everlasting strengthening of the immune device and might hence result in healing successes in problems along with neurodermatitis, allergies, allergies, rheumatism. Spontaneous remedies from cancer have additionally been discovered. It has an anti inflammatory impact, relieves ache and heals wounds, strengthens the nerves and balances the hormonal imbalance of the frame. The remedy additionally has a detoxifying, spasm and shock-relieving effect.

Possible Effects of Reiki

Physical stage

• Pain-relieving and blood circulate-improving.

• Activation of self-restoration powers and strengthening of the immune gadget.

• Detoxifying and purifying.

• Relaxing.

• Pleasantly warming.

Emotional level

• Strengthening of self-self belief.

• Increase in zest for life.

• Release of emotional blockages.

• Relaxing.

Mental level

• Relief from anxiety and pressure.

• Improvement of concentration.

• Liberation from burdensome idea systems.

How Does a Reiki Treatment Work?

A Reiki treatment normally lasts approximately 50 minutes. During a session, the person to be treated lies absolutely clothed on a rubdown table. The practitioner holds his or her arms hands down on or over sure power points at the frame. There are a number of twelve to 15 hand positions which are used in Reiki.

How long the arms are left in every function depends on the go with the flow of energy that flows thru the arms at every factor. Unlike other contact cures, Reiki does now not use pressure, rub down or any form of manipulation.

You can experience the electricity inside the shape of sensations together with warm temperature, tingling, or pulsing where the Reiki practitioner places their palms. Sometimes humans sense the sensations moving at some stage in the frame, at the same time as others do not feel any change in any respect.

There are two kinds of Reiki remedy. One is on-web page remedy, the other is remote. Both kinds of remedy are similarly effective. With an on-website online treatment, you meet a Reiki practitioner in their workplace and immerse yourself in deep relaxation. Reiki is likewise well being! In most Reiki practices, you may be greeted with enjoyable meditation track, soothing scents, and aromas.

An on-site Reiki remedy lasts among 45 and 60 minutes. The Reiki practitioner walks your entire body with their fingers and directs the Reiki electricity into your machine. You stay completely clothed and there's no bodily touch. You only want to take off your jewelry and steel gadgets, as they could hinder the drift of power.

With a distance Reiki remedy, exactly the identical element takes place, best you aren't in the equal room with the Reiki practitioner. Is it operating? Yes! Energy is aware of no space and no time and can be despatched anywhere in the world through the Reiki practitioner. You make an appointment with the Reiki practitioner at a positive time. He or she will be able to do the remedy while you loosen up at home.

Many Reiki practitioners can have a telephone conversation with you after the remote remedy, wherein you could proportion your stories and emotions and manner them together. This is how I take care of my Reiki distance remedies. I will then call you through cellphone or through Zoom to percentage your non-public feelings from the treatment with you and to speak about your modern-day demanding situations in lifestyles. I will provide you with equipment that will help you to carry at the power from the remedy and to assist your well-being. Think of it as an additional 1:1 education consultation.

Both forms of remedy are equally powerful. Many patients even pick far off Reiki treatment due to the fact they feel extra snug in their very own 4 walls and can let pass better there. A Reiki remedy can sometimes turn out to be emotional, specifically while, way to the treatment, pent-up feelings can finally be launched.

What Reactions to Expect During a Treatment?

Everyone reacts in another way to a Reiki treatment. However, many experience the following:

Some human beings:

• Begin to look lighting fixtures and colours in the course of remedy.

• Experience emotional reactions as much as emotional outbursts. Feeling is restoration!

• Feel warm or cold at some stage in the treatment. It may be all around the body or simply positive parts of the body.

• Start to twitch barely or move accidentally.

• Get belly rumblings.

• Fall asleep in the course of the treatment, which is totally ok! The Reiki treatment is still effective - just as if you had not fallen asleep.

• Don't sense something like that and that is also completely normal! You do not always have to sense or revel in whatever in the course of the treatment for it to be powerful.

What Are the Areas of Application for Reiki?

People with diverse challenges find a Reiki practitioner. Be it a top notch loss with deep disappointment, low vanity, family or enterprise-related issues. Some of the patients e-book a far flung Reiki treatment just to deal with themselves - as part of their self-care practice and to loosen up.

Reiki has many areas of application and may be used universally. And I also can say from my many years of practical revel in: yes, it works! And in a superb and gentle way. Just currently I had a affected person who was working difficult on her independence and just wasn't innovative and inspired anymore due to the stress and strain. On a physical degree, this stress prompted her to forestall bleeding. One day after the primary faraway Reiki remedy, she wrote to me that she had her period and that alone relaxed her.

It is essential at this point that I, as a Reiki practitioner, do no longer cause this system. I handiest direct the Reiki power into the patient's body. Thanks to the strength, the body itself then initiates all of the essential processes to regain balance. In reality, it can show up after just one session. Sometimes it takes multiple sessions. Depending on how deep the subject is with the respective individual.

An crucial issue of Reiki is self-duty. Because if you do not dispose of the reason of a particular disorder on your life, the signs and symptoms will come returned. Reiki can do a lot. However, remedy does not relieve you of the undertaking of taking obligation for your existence and nicely-being.

What are the Health Benefits of a Reiki Treatment?

Reiki impacts your complete being. This approach you may enjoy health advantages on an emotional, intellectual, and physical stage. On an emotional degree, a Reiki remedy can release blockages and feature a freeing impact. Pent-up, saved emotions can be launched. You will revel in the deepest rest and stability.

On a intellectual level, a Reiki remedy may be quite strain-relieving. You will be aware that you can pay attention much better and as a result take in statistics more without difficulty. Your thoughts will be cleared and you will be able to recognize and allow move of idea patterns that do not serve you.

On a physical level, Reiki has a ache-relieving effect and may heal wounds more quick. A Reiki remedy is like a detox. All energies that your frame does no longer need are flushed out of the device. After the treatment, detoxing signs and symptoms consisting of diarrhea or tiredness can arise. This isn't a purpose for difficulty, but a completely natural system that promotes the cleaning of your frame. A Reiki treatment additionally promotes blood stream and has an antispasmodic impact. So it's miles a super tool if you be afflicted by duration pains in the course of your period.

How I Discover Reiki Myself

I discovered Reiki due to the fact I'm a traditional over-philosopher. Constantly wondering everything from every angle can become laborious in the end. Meditating is in reality an awesome start to break circling mind and get from your head and into the here and now. I just always felt like there had to be more than that. And it is how I got here across Reiki.

I can be sincere, I become alternatively skeptical in the beginning and wasn't absolutely satisfied that it can surely work. Nevertheless, I approached the recovery approach full of interest and with an open coronary heart and decided to begin the schooling and do the first Reiki degree.

The first degree is the primary building block of the schooling, i.E. The basis. The awareness here is the remedy of your self and others who're physically present inside the identical room as you (as you have discovered, you can additionally do distance treatments). You study that within the 2d degree. After only a few self-treatments, I was capable of put any doubts aside as I turned into greater comfortable and balanced than ever.

So, Reiki is a tremendous tool for folks who belong to the Over-Thinker group. A treatment calms you down on a intellectual level, leads back into your own body and therefore facilitates to ground and attention. I additionally use Reiki on myself for headaches, again and neck pain, menstrual cramps or belly and digestive troubles. If you research this method, you simply have an opportunity tool that can be used in lots of methods.

You also can price your meals with Reiki so your frame can higher soak up and procedure the vitamins they incorporate or your plant life. Yes, you heard that proper! There are experiments that prove that seeds from vegetation which have been treated with Reiki grow quicker than seeds that have now not been dealt with. So Reiki is a actual all-rounder!

I now have all Reiki levels and am also a Reiki teacher. Reiki has emerge as an vital a part of my lifestyles, notwithstanding initial skepticism.

What Makes Reiki Different from Other Healing Methods?

There are two principal differences between Reiki and other recovery techniques. For one component, as a Reiki practitioner, you by no means draw in your very own private strength. You tap into an external power supply. Therefore, you may now not experience tired after a remedy or as if you want to top off your active reserves. On the contrary, because you are the channel for Reiki electricity and it first has to flow via your body so that you can then arrive at your patient, you're taken care of proper away.

On the opposite hand, you may be initiated into your training as a Reiki practitioner. The inauguration is a way of life and Dr. Said to Usui. Only then can you work efficiently with Reiki. The initiation serves to attach you with the Reiki energy and to confide in it.

How Can You Learn Reiki?

So have you ever read this guide and you're like, Wow, I want to learn that? Then the Reiki schooling is proper for you. There are three ranges in total - Reiki Level 1, Reiki Level 2 and

Reiki Master/Teacher. Some instructors subdivide the 1/3 degree and upload a fourth degree for the trainer's degree. You can research Reiki on line or face-to-face. Some persons provide on line training. In particular video instructions, they will train you the entirety you need to realize for the respective degree. You watch the motion pictures at your very own tempo and at your instances. The training is also ideal for busy mothers and experts.

A precise workbook helps you to internalize the content material and way to centered worksheets, promotes your private increase. You get access to a community space where you can exchange thoughts with the opposite trainees. It is regularly the case that there aren't many human beings on your environment who are open to non secular topics. That's why, thanks to the Community Space, you have got the opportunity to share your experiences with like-minded people and connect.

In addition to video instructions, there are stay zoom calls, a welcome call and the ultimate ceremony and live grasp instructions. In the first Reiki diploma, the first master magnificence is ready your intuition and clairvoyance. They will give an explanation for how you may support your instinct, what clairvoyance is and the way it's miles related to Reiki. You will research embodiment techniques to help you connect extra with your frame and address pressure higher.

The 2d grasp class is ready your Reiki guides. Together with the institution, you discover who they are, what you need them for and how you could hook up with them. We perform a ritual collectively. Everything you want for the ritual will be sent domestic on your welcome package deal. These are decided on crystals and formality cocoa.

The crystals should ground you throughout the ritual, at the same time as the cocoa opens and warms your heart; thanks to its treasured vitamins. You can be initiated into the primary Reiki diploma in a 1:1 and on the stop you will receive a certificate. It is a first rate five-week adventure where you will not only learn how to use Reiki but also learn plenty about your self.

Reiki Treatment

1. Stress subside

We have a tendency to nerve-racking up, especially when we are under a variety of strain. The result is often ache in the neck, head or back, but high blood strain or sleep disorders can also occur. Reiki treatment is intended to launch those tensions and break down the blockages of the internal electricity so that you can discover your balance once more. General properly-being can enhance and it is able to be simpler to loosen up on your own. If you experience exhausted and burned out, the treatment will let you get better faster.

2. Sadness and listlessness

If you are going through a length of grief and feel like you may in no way be satisfied again, the laying on of fingers remedy can aid you in this dark time. Reiki is intended to provide you new energy and to make certain that you discover your way again into regular lifestyles in a comforting manner. Quite some people explain that they have regained desire, among different matters.

three. Reiki in opposition to psychosomatic lawsuits

If the doctor tells you that there's no organic reason behind your pain, that does not help you. After all, you sense it besides and you can also be wondering if something is inaccurate with you. Treatment via laying on of palms can produce appropriate outcomes in such cases. Therapists who provide Reiki do no longer rely solely on traditional medicinal drug, but additionally begin wherein it does not know what to do.

4. Relieve persistent pain

Some illnesses reason continual ache. These can at least be alleviated by using Reiki. People who be afflicted by rheumatism or arthrosis specially file excellent consequences. After the remedy, the pain in many of them is substantially less extreme. However, you must constantly recollect that the laying on of arms by no means replaces remedy through the health practitioner. Only in aggregate with scientific remedy can Reiki be beneficial with such painful medical pix and make the struggling more bearable.

Chapter 4: Reiki As A Therapy For Chronic Diseaseas

As has took place in different nations, Reiki is now well known within the West, which includes the USA, its use has spread, even attaining hospitals as complementary therapy in patients affected by ache, terminal ailments or those considered chronic. In this chapter, we want to delve into the concern and permit you to realize the blessings that Reiki can convey to those who discover themselves in those circumstances.

To Complete Therapy

Due to its way of acting, Reiki reaches the complete body, as well as the thoughts and feelings. During the session, the practitioner does not certainly cognizance at the signs or treat only the affected organ or structures, but instead the entire individual receives the benefits. These, via the body's electricity gadget, reach all the ones areas and components that want it. In this manner, the consequences of Reiki could be noticed in any respect degrees, presenting relaxation, accelerated energy, reduction (and even disappearance) of pain, improvement of mood, to give some examples.

It is due to this international motion that Reiki works so well as a supplement to improve the consequences of other cures or treatments, on occasion reaching regions that other methods do no longer attain or aren't taken under consideration.

This recovery of the bodily and emotional properly-being of people who receive Reiki is not in itself a gain, but it additionally brings many extra benefits to the frame.

Reiki can help the immune machine, improves metabolism, can be beneficial in treating migraines or menstrual cramps in addition to intestinal problems which include constipation. It facilitates combat insomnia and sleep higher, will increase attention, reduces strain and absence of power, so it can be an best friend to fight depression similarly to the specific remedy this is needed. It also improves shallowness and is without a doubt useful to live balanced at some point of pregnancy and childbirth.

Improve Associated Pathologies

Many instances, collectively with a chronic disorder, injuries, situations or alterations appear that are not part of the particular symptomatology but that have an effect on the development of the ailment, the nation of bodily and emotional health or the patient's pleasant of life.

Regularly receiving Reiki periods helps to prevent, reduce the effect and even resolve feasible related pathologies without negatively influencing the viable treatment or remedy that is being obtained. For example, it hurries up the recovery of strain ulcers, strengthens the immune device so it will likely be extra tough for health center infections to occur, improves muscle tone in areas with loss of mobility, relaxes and de-stresses regions with muscular overload, minimizes the unwanted secondary outcomes to competitive treatments or medicines, and so forth.

Receiving Reiki Reduces Side Effects

In the case of terminal or unknown cure diseases, the same old treatment is typically palliative, the use of remedy or unique approaches (some quite invasive), to reduce symptoms and try to improve the affected person's pleasant of lifestyles. In this thing, Reiki is a great ally given that, by making use of it immediately to medication, it minimizes the facet outcomes of medicine at the same time as optimizing their healing talents.

In addition, whilst the affected person receives Reiki, his complete body is balanced, the metabolism is activated and the immune gadget is strengthened. Consequently, the character's frame is in a higher position to metabolize, integrate and take advantage of the medication's chemistry more correctly and with fewer poor results.

Reiki Therapy in Infectious Diseases

One of the remarkable qualities of Reiki is the potential to strengthen and prompt the immune gadget. This fact makes it an crucial support in sufferers with severe infectious diseases, with the possibility of chronicity (along with hepatitis B) or that don't have a acknowledged remedy and consequently are considered chronic (for instance HIV). Periodically receiving Reiki sessions turns on the self-recovery reaction and therefore enables the frame combat contamination.

As an example, we need to spotlight a examine posted with the aid of the National Institute of Health of the US, achieved in a residence in Brooklyn (New York) for human beings with HIV and AIDS. The enjoy became executed with people over 50 years of age who acquired and/or had been initiated into Reiki over a duration of three years, receiving weekly classes. Study results showed that T-mobile counts accelerated drastically, individuals described a extra capacity to address addictions, and saw improved wound recuperation, among different effective modifications.

The Importance of Mood

One of the principle limitations encountered by way of a person who has suffered from a critical contamination for a long time or who has an negative prognosis is the emotional disturbance that this includes. Anxiety, despair, worry, irritability, isolation, etc. Emotional states that don't want healing and even boost up the improvement of illnesses which includes most cancers, fibromyalgia or HIV.

Receiving Reiki on a everyday basis enables those humans to sense greater comfortable, to reconcile with the state of affairs they may be experiencing and with a purpose to manipulate all those associated emotions. By improving temper, hormones associated with stress along with cortisol or adrenaline, their level in the blood is regulated. This development within the biochemical state permits the immune system to be reactivated, the frame to be put into a restore nation, the digestive gadget and the liver to characteristic nicely, cognitive abilties, vitality, and so forth. To improve.

Healing the Body and the Soul

Reiki is one of the maximum extensively unfold Complementary Therapies in latest years and identified by means of the WHO. It consists of channeling the Universal Energy of better dimensions closer to the person that is receiving it with the aim of harmonizing and recuperation their bodily, mental, emotional and non secular frame.

Although this is the nice regarded objective of Reiki, its authentic reason is to acquire Inner Peace and Enlightenment or Awakening of Consciousness.

Reiki is the power of radiated awareness and has the traits of the vibration of affection, harmony and restoration.

From colds, gastritis, depression, stress, tension and obese to diseases which include Multiple Sclerosis, Lupus, AIDS and Cancer, it is said that there's no longer any disease that does not have remedy from the factor of view of the Complementary Therapies, a fixed of alternative solutions to standard remedy that has had a boom in latest years within the face of a world this is increasingly more harassed, depressed and full of illnesses.

One of the first Therapies to position itself main this growth turned into Reiki, a system of herbal healing through energies that has been utilized by a few TV celebrities and the HR Departments of important multinationals to improve the nice of life and productiveness of its workers, now not to say the rooms of various hospitals and clinics, wherein we are able to find successful cases of curing sicknesses and relieving symptoms.

Reiki is used as a complementary remedy in Oncology Units to lessen soreness because of most cancers and the facet outcomes of its treatment. In Geriatric Units, it's far used to calm the ache caused by arthritis and rheumatism, further to stabilizing the mood and physical state of patients. On the alternative hand, scientific evidence indicates that humans with AIDS enjoy an development in their immune functions (an increase in T-lymphocytes, for example) after a few treatment sessions.

It is a non-invasive remedy compatible with daily lifestyles, which may be utilized in any state of affairs, because the power adapts to the desires of the recipient. Reiki postulates that with the aid of recuperation the Spirit and balancing our emotions, we will heal our body. That is why inside the long term and as soon as the person has discovered the lesson that this compelled course of studying brings him, it heals the basis of the disorder and stops the advent of different ailments.

It is a very powerful technique to deal with pain, both continual and punctual, because it acts through balancing and unblocking our electricity system, so that our electricity flows more easily to the affected vicinity, helping the body to heal itself from sicknesses, accidents and infections; to conquer states of pressure and temper problems, increase crucial electricity, launch feelings, loosen up tensions, enhance memory, etc.

Reiki works through the direct or oblique imposition of hands to channel power from the Universe to the patient thru their chakras or strength centers, letting them harmonize and balance their bodily, emotional, intellectual and spiritual frame. All that is supplemented with strategies to cleanse the person's air of mystery, their home and place of job, etc. It also can be carried out to animals and flowers or sent remotely or as help in demanding conditions (together with a Grade Exam or a job interview).

Although there is a chain of Reiki Systems created each in the West and in the East from the unique System, the closing intention of all of them refers back to the same goal that captured its discoverer, the Japanese Mikao Usui.

During the Reiki session, the affected person can perceive a sensation of gentle, great and comforting warmth, along side a gradual remedy of ache and a country of deep rest. After several classes, the person typically notices that the comfort is increasingly more extended and frequently changes the behavior that motive the lowering of her defenses. This goes hand in hand with the character becoming the protagonist of their restoration, ceasing to be affected person but as an alternative energetic in this process.

Reiki works even if the person does not believe in it, because it works on a diffused plane and is unbiased in their reviews and beliefs. In addition, it does now not want units, it does now not have contraindications nor does it present any struggle with tablets or different remedies, however as a substitute it has a tendency to lessen the side consequences that they will be causing.

In addition to receiving treatment, each person can come to be a Reikist, no longer always to work as a therapist but to apply this strength to themselves and their cherished ones, on the grounds that it's far a device for private increase that permits the improvement of intuitive skills and increases every day the restoration capacity of those who follow it. It isn't unexpected that more dad and mom are starting this practice every day to assist their little kids sleep and calm their pains.

Therefore, if someone decides to heal and commits himself to this direction of growth and attention, Reiki will surely be a key tool for his improvement. And it would not count what type of Reiki is carried out, so long as it is executed with the actual aim of restoration and coming across that beyond the bodily disorder, there's a spirit this is crying out for help, and that it is time to listen to it.

Reiki Characteristics

• No tough practice or education is required: Once the Reiki channel is open, absolutely everyone can begin to heal.

• The capacity to heal is for life: Once the channel is open, regardless of no longer the use of Reiki, the potential to heal never disappears.

• Empowerment: The greater you operate it, the stronger the recovery electricity turns into.

• No concentration or effort required: The required quantity of Reiki flows automatically and with out concentration or effort.

• Does now not transmit bad power: Reiki does no longer transmit negative power and consequently negative electricity isn't received.

• You don't should agree with in Reiki for it to be powerful: It suggests its outcomes no matter faith or belief, whether or not you consider it or not.

• Effective with the whole thing: Effective for animals, vegetation, things and to purify the environment.

• Complementary consequences with other remedies: The effects are notably elevated by using combining it with remedy or different varieties of herbal remedies.

• Transcends time and area: With the use of symbols, you could perform recuperation at a distance, to the past and to the future.

• Karma Purification: Effective to purify emotional and Karma wounds, and to enhance the genetic records recorded inside the DNA.

• Through self-purifications and meditations, with the vibration of Reiki, it's miles possible to raise the soul.

• There are multiple faculties of Reiki: Usui Reiki, Tibetan Reiki, Gendai Reiki Ho, Karuna Reiki, Tera Mail, and so on.

• Depending at the school, there are three or four tiers that may be accessed, the closing being the Master's diploma.

• It is not a religion, so the person's religious ideals do now not depend.

• The affected person does no longer need to trust in Reiki. He doesn't even need to understand the call of what he is getting. Reiki acts irrespective of the opinions or factors of view of the man or woman receiving it.

• Does not require equipment or gadgets, facilitating its use in any vicinity.

• It does no longer have any kind of war with pills or remedies. On the contrary, it usually reduces facet results.

• It has no contraindications. A Reiki session can not be dangerous.

Benefits

• Treats any kind of infection or physical, psychological, emotional and religious sickness.

• Increases crucial electricity.

• Releases pressure, tensions and blocked or negative energies; stabilizes the mental discipline.

• Prevents illnesses and improves current ones, strengthens the immune system, balances the endocrine system and normalizes blood pressure.

• Purifies and gets rid of energetic and physical pollution.

• Harmonizes the Chakras (strength facilities) and revitalizes the frame, mind, feelings and soul.

• Improves states of emotional disturbance, melancholy, anxiety, frustration, insomnia, and so forth.

• Expands intuitive attention and non secular evolution.

• Improves awareness and memory, frees creativity.

• Enriches scientific treatment, quickens self-recovery.

• It helps us to be happier and to locate internal peace.

• Reiki, contrary to standard medication, not handiest addresses the effect, but additionally the motive of the trouble or contamination (Heal the cause, and the impact will disappear).

• It acts on all forms of cancer, AIDS or other signs and symptoms of immunosuppression and on endocrine dysfunctions, together with diabetes.

• Heals wounds quicker, heals excessive and large burns with out contamination and with out leaving ugly scars.

• Cancer sufferers treated with chemotherapy and radiotherapy word comfort or even disappearance of collateral outcomes and sequelae.

• Reiki can remove from the mind, phobias, traumas, fears, sexual abuse, panic attacks, vanity, insecurity, shyness, addictions, dependencies, anxiety, overweight, and so forth.

• Reiki also can take delivery of to situations related to studies and/or paintings, with the past and the future.

• Reiki power has an innate intelligence and is going anyplace the patient needs it.

• Improves relationships with our surroundings and serves as a tool for private development.

• Reiki is a causal healing gadget to the volume that it allows to align or harmonize the suprasubtle or informatic body of the individual, the shape of their karmas, with the superior fields of religious records of the enlightened thoughts. The Reiki (*) symbols have this challenge, to supply the transformation of character karmic structures that during flip will have an effect on the emotional, mental, energetic and physical states of the person.

• Reiki hurries up surgical recoveries, improves mental attitudes and decreases the poor consequences of medication and different scientific methods.

• Reiki produces advantageous consequences on sufferers, reducing pain, increasing rest, enhancing sleep and urge for food.

You Can Also Perform Reiki

As we can see, with the aid of assisting to lessen the related pathologies and improving the emotional country with regular Reiki periods, the individual feels better and has a higher best of lifestyles. In addition, the body might be extra balanced and in higher situations to cope with the disorder or even sell what's known as spontaneous remission.

One of the elements that have made Reiki any such popular healing device is that you do no longer want to be a doctor, therapist or belong to any doctrine or philosophical present day with a view to practice or get hold of it. Anyone can research it and benefit from it. There are many stories around the world of people with lengthy-term ailments, or who have family in this example, who've decided to provoke themselves in Reiki and perform remedies where and when essential, without financial impact and without depending on all people.

Chapter 5: Teaching Reiki

As there's no clinical proof to substantiate the effective outcomes of Reiki, this exercise need to by no means replace standard clinical remedies. It is best practiced along side ordinary medical remedies. Some sufferers or people may discover Reiki extra cushty than invasive tactics or surgical procedures. For instance, a cancer patient will now not heal from Reiki alone, however it can certainly help them experience relaxed, less burdened and more comfortable. It won't sound like lots, but it is often greater hard to recover from contamination or damage while you can't relax, which I'm certain you can relate to. In this feel, Reiki recovery also can be understood as a coping mechanism.

As said in preceding chapters, Reiki is historically taught by a Master who has been trained via one themself. They then bypass the information right down to the next student who turns into a Master, and continues to pass down the oral culture. At the beginning of coaching Reiki, the Master/practitioner will execute an attunement.

ATTUNEMENT

Attunement, also referred to as Reiju, is a non secular blessing enacted through ritual. The initiation is carried out with the aid of a Reiki Master at the same time as coaching Reiki. By receiving a Reiki attunement, the pupil's electricity channels are cleansed. Once they're unblocked, the scholar is healed through this system. This allows them to experience Universal Energy, and grow to be greater self-privy to the energy within and around them. "The attunement will stimulate the whole bodily, spiritual, emotional and energetic bodies, thereby selling fitness and private increase on all degrees and enhancing the sense of well-being" (Marks, n.D.). You should say that attunement is the middle of Reiki instruction.

Attunement is no everyday recuperation method. The motive Reiki can only be taught via the coaching of a Master is because the actual method of attunement is kept mystery. This is to hold the level of respect among Master and student, and to preserve the sanctity of the procedure. The lack of proof for Reiki can gift quite a few confusion across the practice. It's tough to explain in element the technique of transferring power from one person to every other. The entire thing is based on an man or woman's experience with receiving that restoration power. It's now not something that may necessarily be tested not to mention seen. Reiki is a corporeal enjoy, high-quality understood between Master and scholar. This method that the experience can be and suggest something different from one person to every other. Some of the amazing responses encompass "feeling the energy go with the flow, hearing angelic bells, seeing hues, having visions, sensations of warmth or tingling and the listing is going on" (Marks, n.D.). Also, in advance in Chapter 1 we pointed out the myriad of bureaucracy Reiki teaching can take relying on the practitioner, which creates even extra secrecy and differentiation of the coaching manner. Consistent receiving of attunement is extraordinarily beneficial for the recipient due to the fact one's power channels will regularly be cleansed.

Usui in the beginning incorporated attunement into the Reiki exercise to remind his students in their divine reference to usual power. Attunement is one of the Five Elements of Reiki, and it is through attunement that the expertise of Reiki is given.

The Three Levels of Reiki

There are really hints for coaching Reiki, and that consists of completing the three degrees, or degrees, of Reiki. These are one-of-a-kind degrees of mastery that a pupil must pass with a purpose to turn out to be a licensed Reiki Master and practitioner. As can be predicted, the three levels of Reiki are taught otherwise, however every degree of Reiki education centers on attunement, exercise, and schooling.

Attunement is accomplished at each degree to preserve establishing the scholar's electricity channels and permitting lifestyles pressure energy to freely float in the course of the body. Because they're continuously having their strength blocks cleared, students frequently revel in excessive degrees of self-increase after every attunement. Depending on the teacher or course you take, Reiki schooling can take weeks to months, however the know-how will final for life.

Level I: Shoden

Level 1 is the student's initiation. This is generally the level where they learn all about the records of Reiki as properly. As you already know, this is when the know-how of attunement is first given. The motive of degree 1 is to help the scholar begin to apprehend the way to open their power channels on a physiological level. This stage is concept of as the one in which the pupil learns the way to carry out self-recuperation Reiki on a every day basis. In this stage, the scholar learns the way to channel power through their palms.

Initially, degree 1 attunements were completed 4 specific instances. Some masters nevertheless train this manner nowadays; however, many Reiki masters choose to provide degree 1 attunements in a unmarried session. Because it may be such an severe technique at the start, receiving and mastering to perform attunements can be stretched from at least 12 hours up to 3 months earlier than continuing to stage 2.

Level II: Okuden

Level 2 is where they truly start to understand the attunement extra deeply. Students start working towards Reiki on other people. This is likewise while the scholars begin receiving one of the 5 elements of Reiki: the Reiki symbols. Students use the symbols to invoke the lifestyles pressure electricity on a every day foundation. The symbols are extraordinarily beneficial in acting distance recuperation and sending electricity in other places of the arena.

The attunement in this degree is targeted on establishing the heart chakra. The idea is for students to end up absolutely invested on this process, and they do so with the aid of final their eyes to reduce out all different distractions. Level 2 normally takes six months to a 12 months earlier than the scholar moves on to degree 3.

Level III: Shinpiden

Level 3 is likewise referred to as the "Reiki Master" level. This is as it's historically known as the "trainer's level." At this level, the student turns into a master. However, some college students nevertheless aren't cushty coaching yet, that is why some teachers have a level three that is then followed with the aid of a Reiki Master degree.

Because this is the level where the pupil becomes a grasp, this is why there's so much time among the second and 0.33 level. Level 3 is while the scholar is completely, deeply devoted to Reiki.

The Five Elements of Reiki

According to Reiki Masters and Japanese lifestyle, the belief of "the practitioner is that they don't cause the restoration, nor are they the source of that recovery power" (Bedosky, 2022). Again, the practitioner is merely the channel for electricity. They are unblocking the power that the student or recipient already has within. The practitioner's open channel is available for the recipient to draw strength.

Master Usui taught Reiki consistent with The 5 Elements of Reiki: Reiki Precepts, Meditations and Techniques, Symbols and Mantras, Hands-on Healing, and Reiju. These Elements are part of the machine of Reiki this is used to train and analyze. They connect to shape the path the student will take as they discover ways to use and adapt Reiki via each degree that Reiki is taught.

Reiki Precepts (Gokai)

Reiki precepts, or Gokai, this means that 5 times, are codes used to exercise Reiki. The precepts are on occasion referred to as "Reiki Principles." There are five precepts in total, which Master Usui at the start taught to encourage his college students on their non secular trips. His purpose was for his college students to recite them at some point of their exercise. There are many translations and revisions of the precepts. For instance, Master Takata revised them perhaps to cause them to more comprehensible and relatable for her American students. The following precepts are translated with the aid of a Japanese United Nations professional, true to the authentic Japanese meaning (Miles, n.D.):

Today Only

Do no longer fear

Do no longer anger

With thankfulness

Work diligently

Be kind to others.

The precepts are tenets intended to establish regulation, and can also be used in the course of and for meditation practices. Again, they're supposed to be recited at some point of a practitioner's Reiki practice, not just when it comes to The five Elements for the duration of Reiki education.

Reiki Meditations and Techniques

Meditation plays a massive role in Reiki. Meditation includes getting into a country of peace while the mind continues to be alert. The concept is for your mind to stay present even as with out intruding thoughts. Since meditation abilities like deep respiratory, centering oneself, and searching inward are part of the Reiki process as an entire, the subsequent techniques are gift in the first two tiers of Reiki. In the first level, there may be the Jôshin kokyû hô, Kenyoku Hô, and Seishin Toitsu strategies. In the second level, the meditation approach known as Hatsurei Hô is practiced. All of these techniques can be practiced independently or protected along with your Hands-On Reiki healing.

Jôshin Kokyû Hô

Jôshin kokyû hô is a meditation workout that uses breathing to cognizance the mind. This meditation is grounding due to the fact it is constructing at the Hara, connecting you to typical electricity. This meditation approach to direct you in the direction of "consciously" respiration. Meaning, whilst doing this meditation you are presupposed to focus on the breath in an effort to gradually benefit consciousness of the inner and outer flows of breath. By doing this, you're clearing your strength fields and connecting with the Earth.

Here is an instance of a Jôshin kokyû hô breathing meditation you can practice:

1. First, get into a cushty sitting role. Be sure to ensure your returned is immediately, which means your spine is lengthened.

2. Bring your palms together inside the Gassho hand role. This way that your hands are pressed collectively in prayer, placed in front of your coronary heart.

3. Set an goal for this exercise. For example, In this meditation, I will launch all of the stress I've been wearing.

four. Rest your fingers to your mid-thighs. Slightly lift the middle of your chest.

five. On your first inhale, breathe in thru your nostril and experience that power as it travels from your nostril, thru your chest, and for your Hara (underneath the navel).

6. Hold your breath, focusing on the Hara.

7. Slowly exhale via your mouth even as retaining your attention on the Hara. As you try this, fill your breath expanding at some point of your body. Imagine light radiating past your body and into your environment.

eight. When completed, repeat this meditation for about 5-10 mins. Afterwards, allow your self to loosen up within the grounding energy you've got created for your self.

The more which you exercise, this meditation will enhance your breathing. This makes it simpler to deal with stress as you are gaining manage over the go with the flow of your breath.

Kenyoku Hô

Kenyoku Hô is a "dry bathing" technique. Dry bathing is a cleansing approach recurring. It targets to purify the mind, body, and spirit. The goal right here is to cleanse blocked energy channels. Like the previous, that is extensively utilized to floor you and bring you into the existing moment.

Here is an instance of a Kenyoku Hô meditation you may practice (Shah, n.D.):

1. Gassho—Bring the arms to touch in the front of the coronary heart's center. Hold the purpose to clear anything that forestalls you from being a clean and open channel for Reiki.

2. Breathe in. As you exhale, sweep diagonally down from the left shoulder to right hip.

three. Breathe in. As you exhale, sweep down diagonally from right shoulder to left hip.

4. Breathe in. As you exhale, sweep diagonally down from left shoulder to right hip.

5. Breathe in. On the exhale, sweep down the left arm together with your proper hand.

6. Breathe in. On the exhale, sweep down the right arm with your left hand.

7. Breathe in. On the exhale, sweep down the left arm together with your right hand.

eight. Gassho—Bring your palms to touch on the coronary heart's middle to well known your practice. Cultivate gratitude for yourself and your exercise.

The meditation is to launch whatever that has been blocking your strength channels and stopping you from feeling Reiki energy. It is likewise meant to disconnect you from bad conditions and people that aren't proper on your overall nicely-being. This consists of disconnecting with negative thoughts, feelings, and energy. This is a good manner to put together as you input a meditative state.

Seishin Toitsu

Seishin Toitsu is a mind-unifying technique. Seishin translates to intend 'soul,' 'thoughts,' or 'spirit.' Toitsu interprets to mean 'unite.' The motive is to add goal to the mind so that it will hook up with Reiki. This is a visualization meditation that specializes in constructing and expanding conventional strength within.

Here is an example of a Seishin Toitsu meditation:

1. As before, sit in a cushty function, lengthening your spine. Bring your hands into the Gassho prayer function.

2. On your first inhale, imagine white mild radiating in the course of your frame starting out of your palms, through your hands, in your heart, and all the way down to your belly.

three. When you exhale, consider that white light travelling via your body again, but this time out of your belly up through your coronary heart, fingers, on your hands.

4. Repeat this exercise for five-10 mins. While you do this, visualize your power channels clearing.

5. When you're finished, take a deep breath and express gratitude.

During this meditation, you can sense tingling sensations on your fingers. They might also experience heat or involuntarily move. You must feel space beginning inside your frame as nicely.

Hatsurei Hô

Hatsurei Hô is a method for growing big quantities of non secular power. Hatsurei Hô objectives to unite the thoughts with the body. This method is unique in that it consists of the Jôshin Kokyû Hô, Kenyoku Hô, and Seishin Toitsu techniques. It's also specific because of the phrases spoken, a number of which are the Reiki precepts.

The translation of Hatsurei Hô is as follows:

• hatsu way to bring about

- rei approach spirit

- ho means method

Here is an instance of a Hatsurei Hô exercise:

1. First, loosen up in a cushty sitting position with your spine lengthened. Once once more, convey your fingers into the Gassho position. Close your eyes and produce your consciousness to the Hara.

2. In step 2, you exercise mokunen, which translates to intend 'focusing.' In a low voice, claim "Now I will start Hatsurei Hô." This mantra is also used to conclude this exercise.

three. In step 3, practice the Kenyoku Hô meditation. The reason is to push aside any poor power by means of using contact, even though superficially. Think of this exercise as cleaning your air of secrecy.

four. Move your hands up above your head. Make sure they're retaining in line with your shoulders. Also test to look that your hands are dealing with up and your arms are all pointing towards each other. As you breathe, clear your thoughts and visualize white mild flowing down through your arms and into your entire body. When you get a experience of this Reiki power, begin to slowly lower your palms and fingers.

five. In step five, practice the Jôshin Kokyû Hô meditation. Place your palms face up in your lap as in case you were retaining a tray. Feel the identical white light radiating out of your mind on your middle.

6. Bring your fingers into the Gassho function another time, paying unique interest to your middle hands urgent into every different. Hold this role.

7. In step 7, exercise the Seishin Toitsu meditation.

eight. In this step, you are going to speak the words of the Reiki precepts.

nine. In the last step of Hatsurei Hô, location your arms in your lap once more but together with your fingers face down. In a low voice, say "Now I will finish Hatsurei Hô."

It's acknowledged that this technique is old because it become written inside the book of one in every of Master Usui's college students, Kaiji Tomita, in 1933.

Hands-On Healing

Tenohira "is the act of supporting Ki to emanate from the palms of the fingers for recovery purposes" (International House of Reiki, n.D.-c). We've mentioned this detail of Reiki due to the fact the usage of contact is the maximum commonplace form of Reiki. This is one of the approaches you can heal your self. This takes place just via setting your fingers for your body, or hovering close to the frame. As stated in Chapter three, shifting the ki (life electricity) shouldn't be pressured. Rather, it's drawn via the fingers with the aid of the recipient's body. When the body senses that power, it then takes that energy wherever it's wanted all through the frame. The placement of the fingers at the body doesn't necessarily decide where the strength will float. There are additional elements identifying where Reiki strength is needed, that you'll study greater approximately later.

Reiki Symbols and Mantras

Symbols and Mantras play a massive element in Reiki and meditation as a whole. Symbols translate to shirushi, and mantras to jumon. There are four of every. Three symbols and mantras are taught within the 2d level of studying Reiki. Then, one of every is taught inside the 1/3 level. Shirushi and jumon are used to deepen the knowledge of Reiki by using calling in a particular strength. You may additionally take into account Buddhists are yogis chanting or reciting mantras, and perhaps humming the 'Om' mantra all through meditation. They achieve this to invoke the meaning of the chant and guide them of their exercise. The same is for the Reiki symbols and mantras. The factor is not to call in strength from out of doors of you, but from within.

Remember, all of us have that existence pressure strength within us, and shirushi and jumon can assist summon that power. Additionally, shirushi and jumon permit you to connect with the Energetic System which you will study in Chapter 6.

Symbols

Activating Reiki Symbols

The symbols may be activated with any of the subsequent methods:

• Draw the image in the middle of your palm.

• Draw the symbol with your finger.

• Visualize the image.

• Close your eyes and draw the image together with your third eye.

• Spell the name of the symbol 3 instances.

It doesn't matter which approach you pick out, just make certain you have got a clean aim with invoking each that means.

Positioning Reiki Symbols

After drawing the symbols on your very own palms (or visualizing, and many others.), visualize or redraw the same image on the subsequent regions of the body:

• the recipient's palms or palms

• the particular place receiving treatment

• the recipient's crown chakra

The Power Symbol: CHO KU REI

Meaning: The strength image is used to increase Reiki power. It does so via drawing Reiki power from around you and channeling it to the focused area. Chant the name "Cho Ku Rei" three times. This is an all-purpose image and translates to intend "'God and Man Coming Together' or 'I actually have the key'" (Body Mind Soul, n.D.). The power symbol resembles a coil with an the other way up 'L' placed over it. This symbol may be used everywhere for whatever, together with:

• sealing energies when a remedy is complete

• spontaneous Reiki classes

• growing the power of different symbols

• cleaning bad strength

• helping manifestations.

• periods in clinic or caregiving settings

• for herbs, food, water, and remedy

• for spiritual protection

When used inside the reverse, this image also can be used to name in electricity closer to your self.

The Harmony Symbol: SEI HEI KI

Meaning: This image is used to heal your intellectual and emotional state and sell a feel of calmness. Sei Hei Ki translates to mean "God and Man Coming Together or Key to the Universe" (Body Mind Soul, n.D.). The symbol itself is drawn in a sweeping like gesture and is meant to resemble a wave. The harmony image can be used for:

• releasing terrible vibrations and strength

• supernatural protection

• cleaning blocked energy and balancing the higher chakras

• recuperation trauma

• aiding meditations which will spark off the Kundalini

• helping the removal of addiction

• balancing both the right and left facets of the brain

Sei Hei Ki will help you to repair emotional harmony so you can experience balanced.

The Distance Symbol: HON SHA ZE SHO NEN

Meaning: This symbol approach "The God inside Me Meets the God in You." This symbol may be used to supply a feel of peace and enlightenment. Its appearance is on occasion known as pagoda, because of its tower-like shape whilst the Japanese characters are written out.

• This is the image that could be used to ship recuperation Reiki energy throughout time and area to each person or something. Meaning, this is the symbol you'd use to perform distance Reiki where you send strength to a person no longer close to or who is some distance far from you.

You also can use this for appearing attunements from a distance.

The Balancing Symbol: TAM-A-RA-SHA

Meaning: This image is for balancing blocked strength channels. It looks like a circle that's been divided into thirds with a line on the intersection of the 3 points. This image is beneficial for:

• decreasing ache

- selling grounding strength

- beginning the chakras

The Master Symbol: DAI KO MYO

Meaning: This image isn't in stage 1 or 2, however can actually simplest be used by attuned Reiki Masters. This is the image you will use to heal your or a purchaser's soul. Because it's one of the more non secular symbols, this image is useful for recovery infection and disorder starting from your strength fields and air of secrecy. Visually, it's miles the maximum complicated of the Reiki symbols to draw by hand. The grasp symbol is also for promoting peace and enlightenment, permitting you to growth your instinct and psychic skills.

Mantras

Along with Reiki symbols, Reiki mantras also are a effective way to sell recuperation and balancing lifestyles pressure energy. They are in particular extremely good for cleaning away karmic blocks and recuperation the soul.

- OM SHANTI, SHANTI, SHANTI

'Om' doesn't have a translated meaning however is taken into consideration to represent the sound of the universe. It symbolizes beyond, gift, and future realities. 'Shanti' translates to mean 'peace.'

- LOKAH SAMASTAH SUKHINO BHAVANTU

This mantra translates to mean: "'May all beings anywhere be happy and free, and might the mind, words, and moves of my personal lifestyles contribute in some manner to that happiness and to that freedom for all'" (Murphy, 2018).

- SEI HEI KI

You'll word it is the equal call as one of the symbols. It represents concord and approach "God and guy uniting as one."

- OM MANI PADME HUM

Again, 'Om' doesn't have a particular translation. 'Mani' translates to intend 'jewel.' 'Padme' interprets to mean "lotus flower," and

'Hum' indicates the soul of enlightenment. This mantra is repeated to promote unconditional loving energies and compassion.

These mantras all have specific vibrational energies. The more you exercise with these mantras, the more recovery will take region. Overtime, both the technicalities of the symbols and mantras won't count number as a whole lot as their purpose can be embedded in both you and your Reiki practice.

Reiju and Attunements

Reiju interprets to mean "'accepting/giving electricity'" (Enso Reiki Academy, n.D.). Reiju, as , is also called attunement. Reiju is a ritual where the Master creates a safe area for the scholar so that the pupil may additionally utilize the power as wanted. The Master does so by way of performing an active ritual across the student who would be sitting down for the ritual. The purpose of Reiju isn't for the scholar to receive some special strength. Rather, that is how the student learns to draw in as a good deal power as is needed for his or her specific treatment. Reiki electricity is customary, that means it's abundant. So, Reiki isn't approximately using as much power as possible, but rather it's approximately garnering how a whole lot is vital for restoration. Furthermore, just like the symbols and mantras, Reiju isn't always about getting access to Reiki strength outdoor of you, however about getting access to the energy already inside that is 'hiding' or 'blocked' by using stagnant power. The Master or practitioner is just supporting you see that. They are supporting you recognise your very own potential to faucet into Reiki energy.

Each detail may be practiced by using an character independently, however joined together they provide the practitioner complete understanding of a non secular experience that may be shared with every body thru Reiki.

How Are Reiki and Meditation Related?

Although both practices invoke a experience of peace, serenity, and relaxation, they will paintings together however they aren't always the equal. They are both spiritual practices, however meditation is simply utilized in Reiki as a supplement. Meditation strategies which include deep respiration are engaged to convey both the practitioner and the recipient into an area of calmness in order that they may end up receptive to Reiki life pressure strength.

Chapter 6: Performing Reiki

Reiki may be given by means of every person who has obtained Reiki education. That way which you do not need to work in healthcare or emerge as a practitioner, or be something other than yourself. Above all, Reiki is a self-recovery electricity exercise, and you can stick to self-Reiki in case you select. You can carry out Reiki in practically any putting that promotes a peaceful, relaxing surroundings. When you're sharing Reiki with your self or others, it's now not your energy that you are giving away. You're sharing some time and motivation to help be an energy channel. There's an abundance of Reiki energy—in the end, connecting to Reiki is connecting to Universal energy. So, when you are sharing Reiki, you're virtually simply allowing yourself to come to be a vessel for channeling Reiki energy.

DIRECTING THE ENERGY

One of the reasons that Reiki can paintings without touch is due to the fact power flows in which it's needed inside the simplest course. There are twelve exclusive hand placements a practitioner can use to facilitate the glide of power higher. There are hand placements for your head, the front of your frame, and placements for the back of your body. Directing your hands to positive places can channel the energy there, however the power can also nevertheless glide somewhere else. For example, if you have your fingers on a person's head, they may experience it of their throat. This is to say that in which Reiki is needed, that Reiki will float.

Reiki Circles

Also referred to as "Reiki stocks," Reiki circles began as a way for practitioners to exercise Reiki and acquire Reiki from others as well. A Reiki circle is simply what it feels like: humans accumulate in a circle with a Reiki practitioner, surrounding a person in need of strength recovery. This may be accomplished genuinely as nicely. The factor is that the eye is on one man or woman or maybe an item. As you could believe, as effective as one Reiki practitioner directing their electricity can be, whilst a couple of people begin sharing Reiki electricity with one consciousness, the outcomes may be even greater. This may be in particular beneficial for virtual Reiki healing periods.

Distance Reiki Healing

In a piece of writing for Mind Body Green, Reiki Master, Sharna Langlais, describes the which means of distance Reiki. She states that even as a Reiki pupil is present process schooling, one of the symbols they analyze is the "distance image." When delivered forth, the space symbol allows the pupil to transfer Reiki electricity past time and space. She then goes on to provide an explanation for the which means of this. According to Langlais (2020c), distance symbol facilitates practitioners to open electricity channels in an effort to:

… clean blockages from someone's beyond, as well as carry out reiki on a person who isn't always bodily present. Distance Reiki works in keeping with an historical precept referred to as the Hermetic Law of Similarity, which holds that we're all related, as we're all fabricated from power and part of a bigger entire.

When the Hermetic Law of Similarity is offered on the time of a Reiki healing consultation, the practitioner is able to be part of the recipient's strength discipline. This means that Reiki energy may be sent to all and sundry, anywhere in the global.When Langlais is acting distance Reiki, she will be able to commonly use a picture of the recipient as well as a crystal. Of route, which means the crystal has already been cleansed using Reiki. The objects aren't essential even though, as Reiki may be administered just via "directing mind and strength to that man or woman" (Langlais, 2020c). Amazing, right?

Even Langlais admits to initially feeling skeptical with the ideas of distance Reiki and Reiki circles. However, the extra she educated the simpler it got to create energy connection to humans bodily become independent from her. Once even as acting Reiki over the telephone, her recipient felt her feet tingling. Langlais came about to be sending energy without delay to that location. This has occurred more than once, signifying that long distance works just in addition to in individual Reiki. No be counted the distance, Reiki can nonetheless offer rest, ease, and self assurance.

In a separate article for Well and Good, splendor writer Kara Jillian Brown details her first digital Reiki consultation. She desired to be open-minded, so she agreed to a Zoom Reiki session with Reiki Master Nicole Rutsch. Rutsch practices Holy Fire Reiki, and describes it as an power supply that "comes straight from God, or the universe, or the better energy." She explains this by way of saying that once she channels Reiki strength, it's going directly to the consumer. As said in advance, where Reiki is needed, Reiki will flow. Rutsch says that distance Reiki is so beneficial because the consumer is in their own space, which suggests that it's less complicated for them to be cushty and comfortable.

When the session among Rutsch and Brown commenced, they began by way of turning off their webcams. Brown laid again on her pillows and shut her eyes. Rutsch guided her into meditation. In the meditation, Brown become led through a woodland until she got here throughout a hill. She laid at the hill and afterwards bathed in daylight. When the meditation ended, each Rutsch and Brown have been silent. Brown (2020) tried to consciousness on her breath and when she felt her thoughts wander, she just informed herself to focus:

Instantly, I felt this excessive release in my chest. It was like a ball of electricity erupted and radiated through my frame.

Then it got bizarre. I felt like I changed into laying on a beach submerged in shallow waters and that there was water dashing over me from my feet to my head. Except, the water could not contact me—it simply flowed some inches over me like I was surrounded by way of a few form of pressure discipline. It sounds frightening (specifically on the grounds that I do not like water that a whole lot and can not swim), however it become a very soothing sensation.

When the session ended, Brown felt extremely calm and peaceful. When she described her enjoy to Rutsch, Rutsch defined that in the session, unexpectedly her glass of water tipped. Similar to Master Langlais' session over the telephone, Rutsch regularly "can sense variations of what her customers are experiencing." In a separate experience with a customer, as Rutsch directed electricity toward the recipient's throat, Rutsch began to cough and defined this felt that she turned into flushing out the blocked energy the client had been protecting in her throat.

Brown explains that once consulting with another Reiki Master, Hue Hallums, he says that he's efficaciously accomplished Reiki with people he's had little interplay with in any respect. For example, a patron in New Zealand felt the results of the Reiki recovery power he'd been sending. On the belief that distance Reiki is capable of transcending time and space,

Hallums says, "I recognize that we each have this better stage of self. And so I maintain this ideal photograph in my head, in my mind's eye" (Brown, 2020). In doing this, Hallum says he's directing his attention to the spirit of the recipient.

These studies defined by using Kara Jillian Brown and every Reiki Master is evidential enough to show that no longer most effective does it paintings, however even distantly, Reiki remains very powerful.

Blockages

When you're in track with the physical sensations occurring thru the Reiki, then you may also be aware whilst the glide of Reiki energy stops. This is if you have encountered an strength channel that is blocked and the strength flowing from your fingers can now not bypass freely. When this occurs, don't circulate your hand before everything. Instead simply maintain it in the equal function until you feel that launch of strength. You can also move your hands perhaps an inch or to the left or to the right, or up and down. Sometimes Reiki just needs a touch adjusting for the electricity to keep flowing. Whatever you do, don't leave the blockage. Just be affected person, and wait as a minimum five mins together with your hands in location earlier than persevering with.

The Spiritual Hand

Of route the use of your fingers to manage Reiki should constantly be carried out with the gentlest contact. When placing your palms on the body, there must be 0 strain implemented. When you are deeply attuned, there can be events in which it looks like your arms are sinking into the frame. It's as though something is pulling them into the body at the same time as Reiki is being given. It's stated that that is when "your etheric hand extends itself into the deep tissues" (Désy, 2004). This incidence has been notion of as a signal that your better publications are gift or possibly an angel or Ascended Master. For instance, some have said they feel Takata's presence through the heady scent of plant life.

When you experience this ethereal strength, it's miles likely that the Reiki has transcended to a deeper, religious degree of healing. During this second, it's important to cast off your hands slowly whilst you are completed. Removing your hand earlier than the deep pulling sensation has ceased will disrupt the remedy technique. Remember, electricity flows wherein it is wished. So, in case you experience a tug on your palms, let the power flow as deeply because it wishes to before moving your arms.

Crystals

Although the incorporation and westernization of Reiki wasn't in large part identified until the 80s, the effective power residing in crystals has been used as a source of recuperation for hundreds of years. Shamanic rituals included the use of crystals as they are a shape of Earth Energy (which you may examine more about in the next bankruptcy). In reality, there are many different makes use of of crystals relationship back to the sunrise of time from many cultures. People have additionally been using amulets and talismans for centuries. In reality, substantial ivory beads had been found in a grave in Sungir, Russia from 60,000 years in the past. This might have been in the course of the Upper Paleolithic length. Beads carved from shells and shark tooth had been additionally determined.

Their history dates lower back to Ancient Sumeria, Egypt, Greece, China, and Mexico. The Sumerians used them for magic concoctions, and the Egyptians used them for carving amulets for graves. They extensively utilized them for fitness and protection from night time terrors and terrible spirits. The word 'crystal' itself is the Greek phrase for 'ice.' The Greeks used crystals as amulets to prevent hangovers and for lots other things including maintaining sailors secure while at sea. These uses had been similar to those in Mexico. The Chinese used crystals, specially jade, for musical instruments like chimes. They also made jade mask and beads. Jade turned into visible as the healing stone for kidneys. This changed into additionally believed in South America.

Chapter 7: Chakra Healing With Reiki

During this point in time of latest age spirituality and the mainstream version of Eastern spiritual practices, you probable heard of Chakras manner before you ever picked this e book up. For example, the third-eye chakra and the basis chakra are frequently mentioned in yoga and meditation practices. The chakra machine stems from Hinduism within the historical Sanskrit scriptures, The Vedas. In Sanskrit, chakra translates to intend 'wheel' or 'disk.' Chakras are in connection with the religious factors within the body operating as particular "energy centers"—essential organs and nerve bundles.

Each chakra, or energy center, represents the flow of strength in the frame. Starting from the base of your spine all the manner to the crown of your head, there are seven chakras in overall that run along the backbone. Within every chakra, power is being channeled. So while there are blocks or imbalances of power because of some emotional, mental, bodily, or non secular pressure or damage, the corresponding chakra can not retain to characteristic properly. Since the chakra gadget is operating much like a wheel, this means that while a chakra is blocked, all of the power channels inside us are affected. Whether the strength block became due to an outside or inner stressor, we already realize that any block can purpose even extra minor to extreme outcomes on our properly-being. Because of this it's miles necessary to unblock the chakras that allows you to hold a healthful waft of strength. Unblocking or balancing chakras may be performed without Reiki, however Reiki can be used to energize the chakras. The seven chakras each coincide with physical factors, growing a connection between the frame and the 3 active structures.

THE SEVEN CHAKRAS

1. Muladhara: The Root Chakra

Crystal: Hematite

Color: Red

Element: Earth

Symbol: 4-petaled Lotus and upside down triangle

The root chakra, or Muladhara in Sanskrit, is located at the base of the backbone and is the bottom of the chakra machine for your frame. Muladhara translates to mean 'base.' This chakra is the foundational strength middle, the as soon as that connects you to the Earth and lets you experience grounded and strong. The root chakra represents balance and safety, and is related to conflicts of identification and survival such as economic independence, money and meals. The root chakra derives its power from the earth detail. It's represented by using the color crimson which symbolizes instinctual dispositions, electricity and liveliness. The lotus symbol and the other way up triangle represents the non secular connection with depend and earthly life.

Open: When the root chakra is balanced, you may feel grounded, related, and safe within your frame.

Blocked: When this chakra is blocked, or imbalanced, you may feel physical signs like: lower returned pain and troubles with feet, ankles, calves, knees, legs, hips, tailbone and groin, reproductive and prostate problems, arthritis, sciatica, and constipation. In addition, you can enjoy:

- insecurity

- low self-esteem

- tension

- panic

- worry

- melancholy

- excessive cynicism and negativity

- overthinking

- lethargy

- distrustfulness

- anger troubles

- emotional detachment

- eating problems

- nightmares

A blocked root chakra could be caused by emotions of abandonment, formative years trauma, overlook, economic crises, abuse of any type, and the belief that one isn't safe—some thing threatening your security. A lot of your moves may be due to worry. These fears can take place as paranoid or greed.

2. Svadhisthana: The Sacral Chakra

Crystal: Tiger's Eye

Color: Orange

Element: Water

Symbol: 6-petaled circle and moon crescent

Svadhisthana translates to mean "your personal region." The sacral chakra is located beneath the navel (approximately 1-2 inches). This chakra represents sexual and creative strength and fluidity and is associated with procreation and delusion. This chakra also represents your sense of ardour, pleasure, intimacy and agree with. The sacral chakra is in general linked on your degree of relatability between the emotions of others and your self. This chakra's detail is water that's where the fluid nature of feelings and thoughts comes from. The sacral chakra is symbolized via the coloration orange and a moon crescent with a 6-petaled circle. The circle represents water connecting with the energy of the moon to display the relationship between the moon cycles and glide of water and feelings.

Open: When the sacral chakra is balanced, you can experience empowered, outgoing, and embracing of your sexuality

Blocked: When this chakra is blocked, or imbalanced, you could experience physical signs and symptoms like: lower returned pain, problems with your hips and pelvic location, sexual and reproductive problems, urinary and kidney troubles. In addition, you can experience:

- guilt

- kidney troubles

- poisonous relationships

- bladder troubles

- perception you're unworthy of love

- dependancy

- codependency

- belief that nobody cares approximately you

- obsessiveness/want to control

- lack of motivation

- unhealthy sexual impulses

- decrease libido

- apathy

- lack of confidence

- distrustfulness

A blocked sacral chakra could be because of sexual abuse and trauma. When blocked, this chakra should reason you to feel as if you have no manipulate over your life. You should sense a innovative detachment among feeling judged or responsible.

three. Manipura: The Solar Plexus Chakra

Crystal: Amber

Color: Yellow

Element: Fire

Symbol: 10-petaled circle with the other way up triangle

Manipura interprets to mean "seat of gemstones." The sun plexus chakra is located on your stomach region. It's in charge of your feelings of independence, confidence, power, power, safety and self esteem. It's also answerable for your digestive machine and vanity. Your character and identity are shown right here in addition to self-control capabilities and decision making. The intellect and could also are key institutions as nicely. The shade yellow is indicative of the electricity from the fire detail, related to light power and the sun. The image of a ten-petaled circle and downward triangle is consultant of transformation and progression. The blue in a flame is often proven with a blue hue at the petals.

Open: When this chakra is balanced, you may experience excessive degrees of self-compassion and admire.

Blocked: A blocked solar plexus chakra can show bodily symptoms along with indigestion, pancreas and gallbladder issues. You may experience:

• egoism

• tension

• aggression

• lack of confidence

• feelings of powerlessness

- excessive inner critic

- feeling victimized

- problems with the liver, stomach, and pancreas

- giving up your energy to others

- highbrow problems

- issues assessing the tremendous and negatives in existence

- feelings of helplessness

- fatigue

- manipulating human beings

- loss of ambition

- fear of being rejected

When the sun plexus chakra is blocked you could sense intense bouts of disgrace and doubt. You can be directing your power outward rather than nurturing your very own well-being. You may additionally experience ache or pain within the belly region.

4. Anahata: The Heart Chakra

Crystal: Rose Quartz

Color: Green

Element: Air

Symbol: Two intersecting triangles that shape a 6-pointed celebrity internal a twelve petaled circle

Anahata translates to mean 'unstruck.' The coronary heart chakra is located in the center of your chest above your coronary heart. This chakra is connected to your capacity to like and specific compassion as well as the capacity to acquire each. It's associated with hormone manufacturing and regulates the immune system. It's connected to empathy, reputation, change, recognition and insight, and the capacity to grieve. The shade inexperienced is connected to the heart chakra, and it draws power from the air detail due to its affiliation with the breath and area. The symbols of intersecting triangles are supposed to represent air and its union of various and opposing energies which include male and lady. It additionally links both spirit and be counted. The celebrity that's fashioned by way of the triangles represents connection and concord.

Open: When this chakra is balanced you'll feel a whole lot of joy, love, and gratitude for yourself and the human beings round you.

Blocked: When the coronary heart chakra is blocked, bodily symptoms include: wrist and arm ache, top again and shoulder issues, bronchial asthma, breathing, blood and heart associated troubles. You might also experience:

• loneliness

• no compassion or love for others and the self

• anxiety

• resentfulness/preserving grudges

• disconnect in relationships

• loss of commitment

• incapacity to permit others in

- smothering (of affection)

- jealousy

- excessive defensiveness

- fear of being by myself

A blocked coronary heart chakra can motive you to have problems opening up to others. You may also experience lonely and envious as well. These can be the outcomes of strain, neglect, overthinking, and trauma. Lack of love is one in every of the largest reasons this chakra can grow to be imbalanced and your ability to experience pleasure and inner peace is impaired.

5. Vishuddha: The Throat Chakra

Crystal: Aquamarine

Color: Turquoise/Blue

Element: Space (Ether)

Symbol: 16-petaled circle outdoor of a crescent shape with a circle interior; inside that circle is a downward triangle with some other circle interior it

Vishuddha translates to mean 'purification.' The throat chakra is on your throat. This chakra relates for your verbal or non-verbal communication competencies. It's related to your potential to talk your fact, express your self, and communicate your personal inner power. It's symbolized by sound and the detail of space. This is because while you speak, air is disbursed through the throat sending out vibrations now not simplest heard through sound but also felt at some stage in the frame. The colour turquoise or blue symbolizes this chakra and is supposed to depict the purification of mind, body, and spirit. The symbol of a 16-petaled circle represents purity, the moon, and sound in reference to the ethereal.

Open: When this chakra is balanced, you may sense extra articulate and sincere.

Blocked: When the throat chakra is blocked, bodily symptoms can encompass a sore throat, thyroid and larynx troubles, ear infections, shoulder and neck pain, and temporomandibular joint disorder (TMJ). You may enjoy:

• shyness

• listening to problems

• emotions that you may't express yourself or share critiques

• lack of ability to manipulate your speakme

• lack of listening abilties

• secretiveness

• lack of reason in existence

A blocked throat chakra might also sell feelings of rejection and a worry of silence and being judged. You may additionally have a difficult time finding the right phrases to say a good way to specific the way you certainly feel. These signs may be due to feeling or truely being silenced and that your voice doesn't count. PTSD related to public speakme or expression of emotions is likewise a reason for a blocked throat chakra.

6. Ajna: The Third-Eye Chakra

Crystal: Amethyst

Color: Indigo/Purple

Element: Light

Symbol: Upside down triangle and lotus flower

Anja translates to mean 'perceiving.' The third-eye chakra is placed between your eyes/eyebrows and is responsible for your instincts, instinct, creativeness, information and foresight. It's related to your potential to perceive that that could't be visible or felt. Clairvoyance or psychic skills will also be gift. The light element pertains to the union of all of the factors in their purest forms. Indigo or pink constitute the tender illumination of moonlight. The the other way up triangle and lotus flower constitute understanding.

Open: When this chakra is balanced, you may sense decided and are capable of cognizance.

You also are greater open to receiving the recommendation of those around you.

Blocked: When the 1/3-eye chakra is blocked, physical signs and symptoms consist of: headaches, sinus problems, blurred vision and eye ache. You might also enjoy:

• absence of self-reflection and intuition

• worry of the unknown

• concentration difficulties

• tension

• disassociation with the soul

• disconnection with the thoughts and frame

• clouded notion system

• trouble staying gift

• ideals that what you understand bodily is all there's

• overindulgence in illusions and fantasies

144

A blocked 1/3-eye chakra can motive you to feel or be caused by a mistrust on your own insights and instinct. It can also be due to strained non secular practices and trauma as well as experiencing illusions. You may additionally feel caught inside the daily grind that is existence and may war to visualise some thing specific for yourself.

7. Sahasrara: The Crown Chakra

Crystal: Clear quartz

Color: Violet/White

Element: Divine Consciousness

Symbol: A thousand petals and circles inside circles

Sahasrara translates to mean "thousand petals." The crown chakra is placed in the middle at the top of your head. It represents your connection to spirituality and your dating to the Universe, yourself, and others. It's also related to your lifestyles cause, connection to the infinite, higher cognizance, ecstasy, and liberation. The crown chakra controls your inner and outer splendor and embodies mindfulness. The hues violet and white (the dominant color) in addition to the 1,000-petaled circles are representative of the total moon, splendor, transcendence and renewal.

Open: When this chakra is balanced, you'll experience that you have an unwavering capacity to consider your internal voice.

Blocked: When the crown chakra is blocked, physical and intellectual signs include: nerve ache, neurological disorders, complications, Alzheimer's, schizophrenia, and thyroid and pineal gland problems and issues. You may additionally enjoy:

- memory difficulties

- absence of intuition

- imbalance and shortage of coordination

- isolation

- fear of death

- egoism

- feeling disconnected

- depression

- insomnia

- indifference to the sacred

- disassociation with the frame

- being close-minded

A blocked crown chakra might be the end result of loss of path in existence and the potential to establish and maintain goals. You might also have overwhelming emotions of loneliness because of isolating yourself from others. You may do so out of trouble connecting with others. You might also experience spiritually disconnected.

Opening Chakras

When our chakras are wholesome and open it approach these strength centers are channeling energy in a well-balanced waft. In these times, we experience proper physically, mentally, emotionally and spiritually. However, disconnection with others, injury, or infection can cause these energy centers to come to be blocked, disrupting the flow of lifestyles force energy inside the body. When the strength facilities are blocked, the bodily body factors are affected causing the chakras to become imbalanced and no longer aligned with each other. A blocked chakra prevents us from feeling cushty in our thoughts, body, or spirit, and we're unable to be our first-class selves. We're more pissed off and feature low electricity, and of path this may just result in different problems.

A blocked chakra can occur at any degree of lifestyles. From adolescence to adulthood, our chakras can end up strained via any of our existence studies. For instance, if as a child you experienced forget about or abandonment, you may expand the perception which you are unworthy of affection. In this situation, your sacral chakra becomes blocked and can continue to be that way if now not healed. Later, that blocked sacral chakra and negative belief can happen as dependancy. In some other instance, say later in lifestyles a person develops Alzheimer's; this will motive or be resulting from a blocked crown chakra. These examples ought to even apply to 1 man or woman, as it's possible to have multiple blocked chakra, and one blocked chakra can absolutely effect other chakras as well. This is because of the chakra device operating like a wheel, a flowing active gadget which can't fully perform except all features are balanced and clear.

Your traumas, accidents, and fears can all produce imbalances over a protracted time period on your chakra machine. This can also cause anger, despair, lack of confidence, fatigue and plenty of other problems and demanding situations on your energy device. A compromised strength machine has unfavourable effects to your respiration, self-expression, and ordinary well-being.

This is while Reiki electricity recuperation can advantage you the maximum. As you already know, Reiki is a spiritual exercise, and the chakra machine is the religious connection to bodily points of strength inside the frame.

Needless to mention, Reiki is one of the vital recovery techniques able to cleansing the energy channels. When these channels are cleansed they are open, and this is while you experience your exceptional and are able to relax and experience life. If you're feeling careworn, demanding, indignant or unhappy, etc., then your capacity to enjoy lifestyles and revel in pleasure is exhausted. Aside from the presence of physical symptoms, those are a number of the most obvious signs of a blocked chakra causing your power tiers to be depleted.

Crystals for Chakra Cleansing

You can also have observed that a number of the crystals associated with every chakra correspond with the shade that the chakra represents. This isn't genuine for everyone. For instance, the heart chakra is concept to be represented through crimson for the reason that crystal is rose quartz, when honestly the chakra is represented by means of the shade inexperienced. The way that crystals paintings for the chakras is that crystals' innate healing electricity connects to the meaning of each chakra. For instance, the heart chakra is hooked up on your potential to love, and rose quartz is called the crystal of unconditional love. It's believed to emit intense vibrations of "love, pleasure, [and] emotional recovery" (Stokes, 2021). This manner that rose quartz assists Reiki healing because its very own vibration is the electricity that wishes to update that blocked electricity within the coronary heart chakra.

As stated in Chapter 5, crystals for Reiki are gear used to assist the healing technique of cleaning energy channels. This explains each crystal's courting with the seven chakras. When used with Reiki, each crystal operates like an extra pair of fingers. Using crystals in this placing handiest serves to accelerate restoration with the aid of enabling energy to channel even deeper.

Clearing Space for the Spirit

Remember when you discovered about the religious ritual of attunement? This step in Reiki teaching and recuperation already opens each the crown and heart chakras. The electricity points inside the arms are also activated thru attunement. After a Reiki scholar receives the attunement, their chakras are now open and cleansed, their electricity facilities prepared to be a channel for the recipient. The practitioner's cleansed channels enable them to perform Reiki at the fullest ability. Consider this, from Jacobs (n.D.):

Clearing and balancing the energetic body can growth the vibration of the body allowing a person's electricity to meet the energy of the spirit midway. When this strength is met midway then the person is physically able to maintain communications from spirit. The man or woman is probably in a position to connect to spirit thru sensing presence, physically feeling, listening to, and seeing.

Whether you perform self-restoration Reiki or Reiki on different human beings, having open, balanced chakras will can help you get right of entry to divine existence force electricity. The greater you practice, you'll be able to cleanse your chakras at any time and with faster pace. It receives easier and easier to clear the ones electricity blocks and maintain functioning in a wholesome manner that benefits your better cause.

When your chakras are in alignment, this may particularly help you grow to be greater in touch spiritually as the top chakras (0.33-eye chakra and crown chakra) bring about psychic and intuitive skills. This manner that the extra your chakras are continually cleansed the better your cognizance and greater resonant you're with divine strength and mild. "Reiki works on a religious level as it prepares the body and thoughts accordingly enabling the whole body to put together for spirit. Once your mind and body are organized then you could see greater virtually, recognize with actuality, sense effortlessly, and hear what you need to understand" (Jacobs, n.D.). This method that Reiki is one of the nice approaches you can hop on and undergo a religious journey.

All in all, blocked chakras can reason emotional, intellectual, bodily, and non secular imbalances as well as moderate to persistent ailments. These ailments can motive lengthy-term damage to the frame or even persona if no longer addressed. Perhaps after studying this you could start to notice which you already enjoy signs and symptoms indicating you could have one or more blocked chakras. If you sense that you are imbalanced in a couple of part of your frame, this is because whilst one chakra is blocked, all chakras are affected. Remember, chakra way wheel. This means that the chakras are all part of one machine and that gadget can't characteristic well if every element isn't open and clean of blockages. When there's one imbalance, the other chakras will try and overcompensate for the blocked chakras. This reasons greater damage as all chakras are now overworking, and this could motive them all to grow to be stagnant after being too energetic in this feel. This is all to mention that balancing the chakras is imperative for a balanced thoughts, body and spirit, and Reiki can help restore your strength ranges.

LISTENING TO YOUR BODY

I

t will be difficult to realize in case your chakras are imbalanced or when you have other issues that want to be addressed in case you don't realize the way to pay attention to your frame. Our bodies are constantly in motion, flowing between balanced and imbalanced. Gaining a deeper recognition of your frame is step one in getting to know to understand while there is something wrong. For example, you won't know that your coronary heart chakra is blocked in case you aren't fully conscious that you are jealous or if you're smothering a person with love. In some other example, you gained't recognise that your throat chakra is blocked because some of the structures are more airy which includes being greater shy, secretive, or experience as though you have no reason in life. When you have got that better recognition, you could begin to analyze the indicators and cues that tell you your attention is needed for a certain vicinity of the thoughts, body, or spirit.

SIGNALS

What does "listening to your frame" sincerely imply?

Like chakras, the ideas of "paying attention to your body" and "trusting your gut" have unfold rapidly, however no longer everyone is positive when their intestine is speakme. For a few humans, being attentive to their body is quite smooth, however others battle a bit extra to listen their body's expressions. Sheriff (2019 explains:

'Listening on your body' isn't about intuitively understanding which nutrient you're poor in or which vital oil you need for some thing ailment you're having. To concentrate to your body manner that after your body is feeling some thing, anything, you should truely bear in mind that a signal for something.

Sometimes we feel such things as bodily pains, pain, and so on., and we lessen them to intend, for example, "I'm simply worn-out," or "I slept incorrect final night time," or "It's not anything, it will in all likelihood leave." We try this due to the fact maximum of us are a part of the running class and such things as aches, fatigue, dehydration, stiffness, and so forth., are form of part of our norm. We expect those signs to be the effect of a nine-5 job, or a actual result of just being overworked. Or possibly we experience fatigue and most effective relate it to being overworked or simply no longer getting enough sleep; due to the fact these realities have drained you, you don't truely join it in your feelings, perhaps no longer understanding that your fatigue is genuinely a symptom of a depression you might be going through. Though despair and tension are common, it's now not as commonplace to recognise when that's what you've got been feeling. "Humans also are the handiest species that deprives itself of sleep on purpose" (Sheriff, 2019). These examples can also follow to feelings that feel more wonderful inclusive of feeling fortunate from having excessive strength on an amazing day. Is it absolutely just an excellent day this is bringing you so much strength, or is it some thing deeper? Sometimes even if we're incredible worn-out from lack of sleep or an extended, hard day, we'll stay wide awake for a few greater hours just because we experience it's too early or we haven't checked the whole lot off our to-do list.

Did you ever suppose to recognize what symptoms like fatigue, and ache in reality mean about your physical, emotional, intellectual, or non secular health? Everything you do and experience all through life has an impact, and now and again these outcomes can become cues that some a part of you is trying to tell you something.

What does it suggest to ignore the signals your frame is showing?

On occasion, it can pay off to push your frame and test your limits. For instance, making ready for a marathon run calls for you to be flexible in seeing how far your frame can exert enough energy at the same time as strolling. You do this to peer how a ways you can go and what your limit is, and the greater you educate the in addition you are capable of run. Sometimes pushing via opposition or ambition can produce nice consequences!

Other times, pushing your self too tough has extra poor effects. Not all and sundry's mental, emotional, and bodily health is capable of being driven, and no longer absolutely everyone's internal and outer frame can manage to pay for to exert a lot electricity trying to do so. Over exertion causes nausea, exhaustion and more. Here are some signs you'll be the usage of an excessive amount of power.

• You have luggage underneath your eyes.

• You feel drowsy inside the morning.

• Your hair and pores and skin are dry, such as the pores and skin around your nails.

• You sense fatigued and "out of it."

• You're experiencing stiffness and discomfort in your frame.

• You have a lack of preference to socialize and fulfill commitments.

• You're missing your length.

One of the great approaches to pay attention to your frame is to invite yourself questions. Here are some to hold in thoughts whilst you are aware of over-exertion and exhaustion:

• How do you suspect overworking your body or thoughts is in reality benefiting you as opposed to taking the time to relaxation and recover?

• Are you being sincere about how a lot power you absolutely have to complete something whether it's a mission or a exercise?

• Are you telling yourself that restlessness is part of existence or your routine?

• Do you have enterprise in the way you experience in your body?

• Do you've got manage over how an awful lot strength you are using everyday?

Self-Awareness

The reason of mastering to listen to your body is to gain self-consciousness. To be self-aware is to take heed to your personal character, intentions, desires, and emotions. You are a residing organism residing in a international in which there are consistent outside aggressors like pollutants, strain, UV rays, and so forth.; you are also uncovered to strenuous activities that come along side lifestyles such as faculty, work, gymnasium, or sincerely just strolling, snoozing, and many others. Your mind, frame, and spirit are beneath steady publicity and are liable to something. It's your process to get higher at listening to what your frame is telling you. This isn't easy and it takes time to subconsciously and consciously take care of your well-being on a each day, moment to second foundation.

Part of gaining self cognizance is being able to discern your thoughts, emotions, and behaviors from one another. This approach expertise if the way you're feeling each internally and externally is similar to your actions. For example, being self-conscious manner having the knowledge that fatigue way you need to slow down and get some relaxation. It can also mean noticing which you want extra fiber due to the fact you're experiencing constipation. Self-cognizance way spotting how your thoughts, body, and spirit are reacting on your inner and outside international.

If you're questioning how self-aware you are, ask yourself these questions:

Can you describe, in element, who you're outdoor of the everyday roles you anticipate in life?

Are you able to effectively set barriers?

Are you cognizant of ways the human beings for your lifestyles are responding to you?

Are you comfortable being yourself around others or with yourself?

Do you searching for validation?

Do you pressure over people-pleasing?

Tuning In With Reiki

Reiki is this kind of effective manner to start stepping at the path to self-attention. Why? Because with Reiki you are coming into a peaceful frame of thoughts wherein you could contemplate the sensations you are feeling. "Reiki quiets the thoughts and feelings in order that we are able to get hold of intuitive insights... reiki allows self-consciousness and fortitude to create resolutions in an effort to remaining" (Bertaut, 2016). This manner that through Reiki, you can begin to listen what your body has been telling you all alongside. Self-recognition starts offevolved by means of being able to listen for your body and respond, and cleansed electricity channels and balanced chakras will provide you with the capacity to do so.

Follow the Feeling and Emotion

You can listen on your frame through specially listening to your emotions. We all have six middle feelings: anger, disappointment, joy, disgust, marvel, and worry. Each one influences how we experience, suppose, and behave. For most humans, the very best manner to note what their body is telling them is by means of recognizing how they sense, so it might make feel that feelings are the great way to listen on your body, right? But how do you realize what emotions you're truly staring at? Maybe they're physical including a stomachache, sore throat, or sore shoulders. Perhaps they're emotional like fear, lack of confidence, or anger.

According to Mind Body Green, there are two specific layers of feeling: the one for your frame, which means your inner middle and real nature, and the other, outside psychology that your brain will pay the maximum attention to.

Psychological feelings would be those who occur when your thoughts is jogging rampant gathering a high quantity of facts in an afternoon. This is what can motive worry, exhaustion and more. Thankfully, we've got more than just our minds to assist us locate wherein we're at with our mind, frame, and spirit. In accompaniment with a regular treatment of Reiki those three steps allow you to emerge as greater privy to your mental and physiological country.

Chapter 8: Treating And Healing Your Body

The WHO has accredited Reiki therapy as a complementary remedy for one-of-a-kind health situations, further to different ailments. Reiki is widely used for healing and its effects are very surest. This is due to the fact with reiki the chakras are full of established strength, so that the body gets what it needs at the proper time.

The character who applies reiki, what he does is act as a conductor of conventional energy in order that it reaches the affected person and he can heal himself. In addition, it promotes respiratory and rest. In this chapter, you'll discover treatments on the way to treat commonplace chronic illnesses.

Occupational Therapy

Occupational remedy, which is a part of rehabilitation, goals to improve someone's capacity to carry out every day, self-enough sports, meaningful work, and leisure activities.

These sports encompass easy normal actions (e.G., consuming, dressing, bathing, grooming, going to the bathroom, and transferring from one region to every other, consisting of from a chair to the bathroom or to mattress) as well as more complex normal movements (e.G, getting ready food, the use of a smartphone or pc, handling price range or coping with each day medicine, buying and using).

Occupational therapy emphasizes the coordination of several talents required for even simple actions:

• The potential to experience and move.

• The potential to create and execute a plan.

• The capacity to need to get the activity performed and stay with it to the cease.

These abilties can be impaired in lots of ways. The therapist assesses the patient's wishes with the aid of looking at them in their natural surroundings. He tries to identify potential problems with the social and physical environment. He examines the affected person's domestic for hazards that restriction them from acting an activity. If essential, he then recommends measures to make the home more secure. For instance, hints may want to encompass the usage of brighter lights, getting rid of energy cords in regions in which human beings circulate, or tying cords to flooring. The therapist additionally evaluates the assist that own family contributors and others offer.

Specially skilled therapists can examine a person's ability to power and determine if retraining is needed.

Did you realize ...

• Occupational therapists awareness on supporting the affected person perform precise every day responsibilities that have come to be difficult due to a sickness or injury.

• Many specialised gadgets, along with grasping aids and massive-handled utensils and tools, can help a patient characteristic.

Patients with impairments work with the occupational therapist to perceive and prioritize their desires and decide suitable tactics and sports. If a affected person has issues managing cutlery, therapy can encompass physical activities that promote first-class motor skills, e.G. Insert pins right into a breadboard. A reminiscence sport can educate recognition and retrieval. Adaptive techniques can help the patient to apply his strengths to make amends for his impairments. For example, a patient with a paralyzed arm may also analyze new methods to get dressed, tie your shoes or button. As you development, the obligations turn out to be greater challenging.

Auxiliary Devices

Occupational therapists propose gadgets that promote the patient's independence (assistance devices). Therapists show patients how to use the gadgets and if important, assemble or modify specific devices. These devices encompass the subsequent:

Orthotics are gadgets that stabilize damaged joints, ligaments, tendons, muscle tissues and bones. Most orthoses are tailored to the desires and anatomy of the patient. Orthoses are regularly utilized in footwear. They shift the man or woman's weight to exceptional regions of the foot to compensate for lost characteristic and prevent malfunction from taking place. They additionally assist to help the frame weight, alleviate ache and offer help. The therapists can both assemble and adapt those orthoses. Orthoses are regularly very costly and aren't blanketed through insurance.

Splints may be used to save you joints from remaining in a flexed function. When sufferers can't circulate a limb usually (e.G., in the event that they have arthritis or are paralyzed after a stroke), the limb frequently bends slightly and remains in that role. With the assist of splints that keep the limb in a directly position, it is feasible to prevent the joint from freezing in a sure role.

Crutches encompass walkers, crutches, and canes. They assist the affected person to aid their body weight and balance. Each device/product has its advantages and disadvantages and is to be had in distinctive fashions. Occupational therapists can assist patients pick the walker that is maximum suitable for them.

Wheelchairs allow patients who cannot walk to get from A to B. Some self-propelled models are very solid. These models allow the patient to ascend and descend over choppy terrain or curbs. Other fashions are designed to be pushed by way of a 2nd person. These models are much less stable and slower.

Mobility scooters are battery powered carts on wheels with a steerage wheel or tiller take care of. They have velocity control and might force backwards and forwards. Scooters are suitable for riding on company, instantly terrain outside and inside homes, however cannot pass up or down stairs or curbs. They are useful for sufferers who can most effective stand for brief periods of time or most effective walk short distances, e.G. To and from the mobility scooter.

Prostheses are synthetic frame components, generally limbs. For example, for a patient with an amputated arm, the therapist might also propose an synthetic arm (prosthesis) that has forceps to preserve objects. Most occupational therapists can teach sufferers with amputated limbs to use their synthetic limbs or different devices to higher perform their daily duties.

Physical Therapy

Physical remedy, a factor of rehabilitation, includes workout and manual operating of the body with an emphasis at the back, upper fingers, and legs. It can be used to enhance joint and muscle feature. The affected person can stand extra stably again, maintain his stability, walk and climb stairs. The measures include:

• Exercises to increase range of movement.

• Exercises to reinforce the muscular tissues.

• Coordination and stability physical games.

• Walking training.

• General conditioning sporting activities.

- Transfer schooling.

- Exercises with a tilting table.

Exercises to Increase Range of Motion

After a stroke or extended mattress relaxation, the range of movement is commonly constrained. Limited range of motion can cause ache, affect someone's ability to function, and increase the danger of pores and skin rashes and stress sores. Range of motion tends to lower with age, although this improvement does not save you healthy older people from looking after themselves.

Before beginning remedy, therapists regularly assess variety of movement using an device referred to as a goniometer, which measures the maximum angle of movement of a joint. The therapist also determines whether the motion restrictions are resulting from stiff muscles or stuck ligaments and tendons. If the muscle tissues are stiff, the joint can be stretched more. In the case of bonded ligaments and tendons, the joint must be stretched lightly, and surgical procedure is on occasion required earlier than range of motion may be multiplied. Stretching sports are greater effective and less painful if the tissues were warmed up beforehand. Therefore, the therapist applies warmness first.

Range of motion sports are categorised into three kinds:

• Active sports: These sporting events are appropriate for people who can educate a muscle or joint unaided. They should circulate their limbs on my own.

• Actively Assisted Exercises: These sports are appropriate for those who can flow their muscular tissues with a little assist and those who can flow their joints with pain. People pass their limbs on their own, however receive help from the therapist (manually, with bands, or different gadgets).

• Passive sports: These physical games are suitable for individuals who are not able to actively participate in the exercises. You do not should do whatever. The therapist movements their limbs to save you, among different matters, contractures (everlasting stiffening of muscle tissues as a result of loss of exercising).

Actively assisted and passive variety of movement sports are performed lightly to avoid injury. Occasionally, those sporting activities also can be uncomfortable to a point.

The affected joint is moved beyond the pain factor, but there ought to be no lingering pain after the workout is entire (pain that lasts after the motion is stopped). Longer, mild stretches are extra powerful than short, difficult ones.

Exercises to Strengthen the Muscles

Many physical activities boom muscle power. All are regularly multiplied in resistance. If a muscle could be very weak, shifting in opposition to gravity is sufficient. As muscle tissues emerge as stronger, resistance is progressively elevated thru using latex bands or weights. This will increase muscle mass and energy even as also enhancing patience.

Coordination and Balance Exercises

These sporting activities can assist patients who've coordination and stability issues, most typically caused by stroke or mind harm. Coordination sporting activities are intended to assist sufferers to address certain tasks. These sporting activities contain repeating a meaningful motion that works extra than simply one joint or muscle, consisting of picking up an object or touching a frame component.

Balance sporting events are to begin with achieved the usage of parallel bars at the same time as the therapist stands at once at the back of the affected person. The individual shifts the weight from the proper to the left leg with rocking actions. Once this workout may be completed accurately, the load can be shifted from front to returned. Once those physical activities are mastered, the affected person can carry out the sporting events with out the double bars.

Walking Exercises

Walking with or without assist can be the main goal of a rehabilitation program. Before starting gait sporting events, sufferers have to be able to preserve their balance even as status. To enhance stability, the patient normally stands among parallel bars and shifts the weight backward and forward and front to returned. For protection, the therapist stands directly in front of or in the back of the patient. Some human beings need to increase their joint mobility or muscle energy earlier than they can start strolling physical activities. Other sufferers require an orthopedic resource, such as a corset.

As quickly because the affected person is ready for gait sporting events, those can first take place on double bars after which be persevered with mechanical aids which include a on foot resource, crutch or cane. Some patients need to wear a unique harness that lets in the therapist to ward off falls.

As quickly because the patient can thoroughly stroll in a immediately line, overcoming curbs and mountaineering stairs are practiced. When going up stairs, the sound (properly) leg is used first. When descending the stairs, the affected (awful) leg is used first. The adage desirable is up, horrific is down can serve as a useful reminder. Family individuals and caregivers who help the affected person to stroll should learn to do so well.

General Conditioning Exercises

A mixture of mobility, muscle constructing and on foot sporting events is used to counteract the effects of prolonged bed relaxation or immobilisation of limbs. General conditioning sporting activities enhance cardiovascular fitness (the potential of the coronary heart, lungs, and blood vessels to supply oxygen to operating muscle tissue), preserve and improve flexibility and muscle electricity.

Transfer Training

For many patients (specifically after a hip fracture, amputation or stroke), transfer schooling is an critical rehabilitation purpose. Safe and unbiased motion from bed to chair, wheelchair to lavatory, or chair to a standing role is extremely important to allow the affected person to stay at domestic. Patients who can't make this switch without outside help generally require round-the-clock care. The caregiver can assist the affected person to perform the transfer with a walking or posture belt.

The methods utilized in transfer education depend upon the subsequent circumstances:

• Whether the affected person can endure weight on one or each legs.

• Can he keep his balance correctly?

• Is he paralyzed on one aspect?

Assistive gadgets can sometimes be used to assist. Patients who have trouble transitioning from sitting to status may also advantage from a seat crane or a chair with an elevated seat.

Tilting Table

After numerous weeks of strict bed relaxation or a spinal twine damage, a affected person's blood stress may additionally drop rapidly after they stand up, and they may experience dizzy. A tilting table can help the affected person in this example. This manner can help slim or widen the blood vessels depending at the response to postural changes. In this way, the blood pressure can be balanced when converting position. The patient lies supine on a padded desk with a footrest and is supported by way of a belt. The table is tilted very slowly, relying on how nicely the patient tolerates it, until the affected person is almost upright. By slowly changing posture, the vessels learn to constrict once more. The duration of time the patient stays within the upright function relies upon on their tolerance of the location, however should no longer exceed 45 mins.

The tilting table is used once or twice an afternoon. Its effectiveness varies and relies upon on the type and degree of impairment.

Stroke

When you have a stroke, the arteries that deliver your brain end up blocked or ruptured. This reasons brain tissue in part of the mind to die (cerebral infarction) and signs and symptoms seem very abruptly.

• Most strokes are ischemic (because of blockage of an artery) and some are hemorrhagic (caused by rupturing of an artery).

• Transient ischemic attacks are much like ischemic strokes, except that permanent mind harm does not arise and signs are reversible inside an hour.

• Symptoms come on and may consist of muscle weak spot, paralysis, uncommon sensations or lack of sensation on one aspect of the body, difficulty speakme, confusion, blurred imaginative and prescient, dizziness and lack of balance and coordination, and inside the case of a hemorrhagic stroke, intense, sudden complications.

• Diagnosis is primarily based by and large on symptoms, but imaging and blood assessments are also accomplished.

• Recovery from a stroke depends on many factors, such as the region and quantity of mind damage, the individual's age, and the presence of other medical situations.

• Controlling high blood strain, excessive ldl cholesterol, and excessive blood sugar, and quitting smoking can assist save you strokes.

• Treatment may additionally consist of drugs that make blood less probable to clot or break up clots and now and again diverse procedures to deal with blocked or narrowed arteries, or surgical operation to dispose of a blood clot (such as angioplasty).

A stroke is a cerebrovascular disease as it includes the mind (cerebro) and the blood vessels (vascular) that supply blood to the mind.

The blood deliver to the mind

The mind is provided with blood via pairs of massive arteries:

• The inner carotid arteries bring blood from the coronary heart inside the the front of the neck to the mind.

• The vertebral arteries that deliver blood from the heart via the neck.

In the skull, the vertebral arteries unite and shape the cranial artery (in the back of the head). The internal carotid arteries and the cranial artery divide into numerous branches, together with the cerebral arteries. Some branches form a circle of arteries (Willis circle) that join the vertebral arteries and internal carotid arteries. Other arteries branch off this circle of Willis like roads from a roundabout. These branches carry blood to all regions of the brain.

When the big arteries imparting the brain grow to be blocked, some human beings haven't any symptoms or just a moderate stroke. However, other people with the same blockage have a huge ischemic stroke. Why? Part of the reason lies within the collateral arteries. Collateral arteries run among other arteries and make additional connections. The Willis circle and the connections between the arteries that branch off from it are examples of these arteries. Some human beings are born with huge collateral arteries that could guard them from strokes. When an artery becomes blocked, blood maintains to flow through a collateral artery, occasionally stopping a stroke. Some human beings are born with small collateral arteries.

The frame can also guard itself from strokes with the aid of forming new arteries. When blockages increase slowly and step by step (as in atherosclerosis), new arteries can develop in time to supply blood to the affected place of the brain, therefore preventing a stroke. If a stroke has already happened, new arteries can help save you a 2nd stroke (however can not opposite the harm that has already happened).

Stroke is the world's second main reason of loss of life. In the USA, stroke is the 5th main purpose of dying and the main purpose of disabling apprehensive machine damage in adults. Each 12 months, about 795,000 human beings within the United States be afflicted by a stroke. Approximately one hundred thirty,000 human beings die from a stroke.

.